MW00451933

Narkomania

Narkomania

Drugs, HIV, and Citizenship in Ukraine

Jennifer J. Carroll

Cornell University Press

Ithaca and London

Copyright © 2019 by Cornell University

All rights reserved. Except for brief quotations in a review, this book, or
parts thereof, must not be reproduced in any form without permission in
writing from the publisher. For information, address Cornell University
Press, Sage House, 512 East State Street, Ithaca, New York 14850.
Visit our website at cornellpress.cornell.edu.

First published 2019 by Cornell University Press

Librarians: A CIP catalog record for this book is available from the
Library of Congress.

ISBN 9781501736919 (cloth)
ISBN 9781501736926 (pbk)
ISBN 9781501736933 (pdf)
ISBN 9781501736940 (epub/mobi)

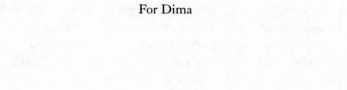
For Dima

If we, social scientists, took stock of the problems we have solved for humanity, would we have reason to be proud? ... When did we ever stop human suffering on such scales as witnessed in Iraq and Afghanistan—or on any scale, for that matter? What did we ever do to stop this or any war?

MARK DE ROND, *DOCTORS AT WAR*

Contents

ILLUSTRATIONS

Preface

Ethnography relies on trust. Long-term engagement with the communities in which we live and work is a hallmark of ethnographic research, the goal of which is to cultivate mutual trust between us and those from whom we hope to learn. We begin our research with much to prove. We must assure our funders that we can get the job done, demonstrate our commitment to serve the communities we live in, and convince our informants that we are not complete idiots. Other anthropologists I know have had to learn skills like flipping sheep on a farm, sweet-talking police at the train station, and canning vegetables in a bathtub before their hosts would take their overtures seriously. In my own experience, even knowing the right way to ask for a check or call out a stop to the bus driver makes an enormous difference in the amount of trust that people are willing to afford you. Because, no matter where you are in the world, once the initial hospitality dies down, the fact that you can be a nuisance bears more and more weight on your social interactions. People won't want to talk to you if you clearly don't know what you're doing.

Ethnography also requires trust between the researcher and the audience she is writing to. This, too, is something to be earned. It comes not only from the experience and expertise that the ethnographer offers through her writing but also through her capacity to present what she has learned through her research as a real, authentic, and (above all) believable slice of the human experience. Achieving this latter goal can be particularly hard when writing about the lives of people who use drugs because, as an early reviewer of my work once observed, "Everyone knows that addicts lie." I do not adhere to this view, of course. I have had the great privilege of meeting numerous intelligent, complicated, fascinating people over the course of my research. They have shared life stories with me and recounted intimate personal details. They have tutored me in the ways of their many worlds. They have given freely of their time and emotion to teach me their philosophies and listen to my own. Some of them have also used drugs. These individuals do not stand out, either in my data or in my memory, as particularly "different" kinds of humans.

Yet presenting informants who use drugs as the complex human beings I know them to be has occasionally given readers cause to distrust what I write. It has been suggested, at one time or another, that I glorify drug use, that I present a deceptively rosy picture of lives that include drug use, and that I have been deceived by my own informants, taken in by the web of lies they spun so that I saw only what they wanted me to see, not things as they really were.

Perhaps you, reader, will feel this way. Perhaps drug use has touched your life. Perhaps you have struggled with substance use disorder. Perhaps you have watched a loved one in the midst of that struggle. Perhaps that struggle has taken loved ones from you. If this is your experience, know that I, too, am familiar with this pain. Know that you, and only you, are the owner of your experiences and that this book cannot, and does not seek to, speak back to them in anyway. I do not wish to tell you your story. But in the interest of being an ethnographer worthy of your trust, I would like to tell you mine.

As a college student in Portland, Oregon, I began making regular visits to a city-sanctioned tent camp that had approximately sixty residents. What began as a class project developed into several lasting friendships with community leaders in the camp. Over the next few years, I would regularly bring high school groups to the camp to visit, serve a community meal, and get to know the residents. Around this time, I also became involved with a local youth shelter, spending one or two shifts per week in their kitchens helping to train other, new volunteers to be effective allies for the youth who used these services. This youth shelter also offered a community medical clinic and syringe access program. Wanting to learn more about the impact of these services, I began taking weekly shifts in the program, where I ended up serving for nearly two years. During this time, I learned a great deal about common injection practices, the risks faced by program participants, and the concerns they managed on a daily basis.

I moved to Chicago a few years after graduation and, there, was taught about the overdose-reversing drug naloxone by Dan Bigg, the co-founder of the Chicago Recovery Alliance (CRA). In addition to pioneering naloxone distribution in the United States (a true revolution in public health now acknowledged as a core strategy for overdose prevention), Dan and his team members endorsed a program of compassion and personal empowerment for CRA participants. It is hard to overstate the enormity of the impact Dan left on me and on so many others. Since leaving the Texas church in which I was raised, Dan was the only person I had yet met in my young adult life who preached a gospel of fierce and unconditional love for all people. I think he was the first person in many of our lives who was willing to loudly and shamelessly declare that people who use drugs are valuable, deserving persons—even when it put his reputation and his livelihood at risk. When he passed away suddenly in August 2018, a tidal wave of grief swept over the harm reduction community. When I received the news via text message, I couldn't catch my breath. I pulled my car off the road and wept.

In 2007, I earned a master's degree at Central European University. My thesis research took me to Odessa, Ukraine, where I shadowed outreach workers from a local harm reduction organization and syringe access program. Most of the individuals I shadowed were, themselves, receiving daily doses of methadone to treat their opioid use disorder. Thanks to the openness and generosity of these individuals, I learned a great deal about how these programs I came to know in the United States could be adapted to serve people with different needs in a very different kind of community. Over the next several years, I would clock hundreds of hours accompanying people engaged in this kind of outreach across Ukraine, meeting more program participants than I could count and getting to know a few of them very well.

In 2010, the scope of my research in Ukraine expanded. I began systematically interviewing medical providers who served people who use drugs in HIV hospitals, tuberculosis hospitals, and narcology clinics. I also began interviewing and collecting life histories from the patients receiving treatment for opioid use disorder in these spaces. I spent my days in the courtyards and waiting areas of various local hospitals. Over time, I developed friendships with many of the individuals receiving care. This kind of intimate work among people deeply affected by substance use was nearly all I did from late 2012 to early 2014.

When I returned to the University of Washington in 2014 to complete my PhD, I began working with the People's Harm Reduction Alliance (PHRA), a "peer-run" harm reduction organization based in Seattle, Washington. In practical terms, their "peer-run" moniker meant that at least 51 percent of their board and 51 percent of their regular volunteers had to self-identify as someone who uses drugs. During my time with PHRA, I learned a great deal about the evolving drug market in the United States, about the effects of drug policy on the individuals that PHRA serves, and about how difficult it can be for politically active and well-organized social advocates who also happen to use drugs to find community partners whom they can trust. I also saw firsthand how challenging it can be to offer effective, evidence-based public health services when much of the surrounding community despises the people you are hoping to serve.

The people of PHRA came to feel like family. They were young kids and old folks. Some were living on the street. Some were students in my university classes. Some were gruff, rude, and tired, but most were warm and genuine and put energy into building loving relationships with each other. We sang for birthdays. We celebrated weddings and births. We grieved when someone passed away. Despite everything PHRA was doing to keep the community safe, we nevertheless held more memorials than we did celebrations. That is precisely the reason why we never gave up that work.

In 2015, I joined the faculty of Brown University as a postdoctoral fellow in the medical school. There, I was recruited by the cochairs of the Rhode Island Governor's Overdose Prevention Task Force to develop and implement an ethnographic research protocol to monitor the effects of new drug control and overdose prevention policies rolling out across the state. From 2015 until 2017, this work kept me involved on a near daily basis in the lives of individuals who use opioids in Rhode Island. My work took me to syringe access programs, day centers for men and women engaged in commercial sex work, open air drug markets in parking lots and bus malls, methadone clinics, pain clinics, and late-night emergency rooms. The people of Rhode Island generously welcomed me into their lives, debriefing with me after accidental overdoses, sharing strategies for helping each other stay "straight," and collectively grieving for the devastating number of loved ones who had died from accidental overdose since fentanyl entered the drug supply in 2013.

In 2017, I began working with the nation's largest federally funded interdisciplinary opioid overdose prevention effort. I was brought into this project—a collaboration between the High Intensity Drug Trafficking Areas (a program of the Office of National Drug Control Policy) and the National Centers for Disease Control and Prevention—to serve as an expert and scientific adviser on substance use, strategies for overdose prevention, and the public health effects of drug policy. As a consultant, I am able to share the wealth of knowledge I have gained from my nearly two decades of living and learning in the worlds of substance use with state and local leaders working in government, law enforcement, and public health. I recognize that gaining this knowledge and sharing it with this audience are both privileges that I am exceedingly fortunate to have been granted. Out of humility and gratitude for those privileges, I do my very best to report honestly the things I have seen, to show the good and the bad together as we experience them in real life.

As I was writing this book and pondering this preface, Dan Hirschman, a friend, sociologist, and fellow Brown faculty, brought to my attention the prologue of another, very different text: W. E. B. Du Bois's *Black Reconstruction in America*. In his note, "To the Reader," Du Bois writes:

> It would only be fair to the reader to say frankly in advance that the attitude of any person towards this story will be distinctly influenced by his theories of the Negro race. If he believes that the Negro in America and in general is an average and ordinary human being, who under given environment develops like other human beings, then he will read this story and judge it by the facts adduced. If, however, he regards the Negro as a distinctly inferior creation, who can never successfully take part in modern civilization and whose emancipation and enfranchisement were gestures against nature, then he will need something more than the sort of facts that I have set down. But this latter person, I am not trying to convince. I am simply pointing out these

two points of view, so obvious to Americans, and then without further ado, I am assuming the truth of the first. In fine, I am going to tell this story as though Negroes were ordinary human beings, realizing that this attitude will from the first seriously curtail my audience. (Du Bois 1998)

Suffice to say that little is to be gained from comparing the general situation of people who use drugs today to the plight of as many as ten million people who emerged from generations of violent captivity only to continue fighting for their right to live and be free in the midst of those who once held them captive. But, to the degree that Du Bois has tapped into something fundamentally human in his observation, this passage can be instructive in telling us how our reactions to texts, like the one contained in this book, may be informed by our previously held dispositions toward the subject at hand.

In this book, my aim is to tell the stories that I and others have lived through as honestly as possible. Rather than vilifying or glorifying various choices made by the people I have known, I try to present decisions and behaviors of all kinds as fundamentally human, as reflective of loves, desires, and fears that, at some level, we all share. As with all ethnography, I hope to earn your trust as you read through these pages. Good ethnography relies on trust; at the same time, our perceptions of what is "true" often bend to meet our preconceived beliefs and experiences. So, while I cannot promise that everything you read will ring true, I can tell you, with confidence and sincerity, that this is how it all really happened.

ACKNOWLEDGMENTS

I am deeply indebted to many individuals and institutions for their support of this project. First among these is the faculty in the Department of Anthropology at the University of Washington, who provided unwavering support as I, a complicated individual, navigated my way through a complicated project in a challenging political climate. I am grateful especially for the guidance and leadership of Laada Bilaniuk and Janelle Taylor, who performed the significant work of holding me to high standards both in my academic endeavors and in the dignity and professionalism with which I have carried them out. I am equally grateful to Jared Baeten, who enthusiastically made way for my learning and professional development in an institution that didn't always know what to do with me. He has done more than he can possibly know to instill confidence and humility in me in equal measure.

Much of this book was written while I was a postdoctoral fellow in the school of medicine at Brown University. Tim Flanigan was instrumental in affording me this opportunity, and he put significant work into my professional development as a clinical as well as an ethnographic researcher. Jody Rich and Traci Green have also graciously involved themselves in my research career. I consider all of them mentors, colleagues, honorable coconspirators, and friends. While at Brown, I received support from the Brown Ukraine Collaboration, a joint venture between the Brown University Center for AIDS Research and health-service providers working in the area of infectious disease in Ukraine through the support of the Elena Pinchuk ANTIAIDS Foundation. This collaboration facilitated follow-up work in Ukraine, which was essential for the completion of this book, and kept me in close collaboration with many talented and deeply committed scholars, both American and Ukrainian, working to improve public health in Ukraine.

Much of the work included in this book was presented at academic conferences and further developed in the fine company of many scholars who invested themselves in my scholarship and provided mentorship and guidance at various stages of this process. In this vein, I especially want to acknowledge Eugene Raikhel, Dominique Arel, Erin Koch, Mayhill Fowler, Sarah Phillips, and Michael Kennedy. I am equally grateful to Sarah Besky, Tomas Matza, Elizabeth Dunn, and Jason De Leon, who offered time and energy to this project and provided blunt, thoughtful, exceedingly helpful advice in clearing various logistic and professional hurdles along the way. An extra dose of gratitude goes to Jason for the truly absurd level of enthusiasm he has displayed for this project and for the advancement of my career in general. Buddy, I appreciate you so much, you don't even know.

I have been extremely fortunate to belong to a community of peers working in Eastern Europe for many years. This group has been a constant source of energy, camaraderie, mutual support, collaboration, and joy. It includes, in no particular order, Emily Channel-Justice, Deborah Jones, Jennifer Dickinson, Elizabeth Peacock, Heidi Bludau, Michael Rasell, Erin Koch, Jonathan Stillo, Jessica Robbins, William Risch, Tom Junes, Mayhill Fowler, Maryna Bazylevych, Zane Linde-Ozola, Lauren Rhodes, Tatiana Chudakova, Shelly Yankovskyy, Monica Eppinger, Oleh Kotsyuba, Larisa Kurtovic, Tanya Bulakh, Iryna Koshulap, Jessica Zychowicz, Sabina Stan, and many more whom I will surely be kicking myself in days to come for not mentioning here. You all have, very literally, been my sanity and my rock in more ways than I could possibly describe.

I would be remiss if I didn't make special mention of the profound influence that Kasia Bartoszynska has had on me as a friend and as a role model.

Words cannot do justice to the love and support she has provided in the time I have known her. I consider myself blessed to be in her orbit. Countless thanks, also, go to Ligaya Beebe, Sean Thomson, Peter McMahan, Harold Gabel, Gemma Petrie, and Erik Cameron who all insisted that I was able to accomplish this thing, even when I didn't believe it myself.

My fieldwork in Ukraine was supported, at various stages, by Foreign Language and Area Studies (FLAS) fellowships, provided by Title VI funds from the U.S. Department of Education; the International Research and Exchanges Board (IREX) Title VIII Embassy Policy Specialist Program; and a Doctoral Dissertation Research Grant from the Wenner-Gren Foundation. My work in Ukraine could not have been accomplished without the support and assistance of Jim Davis, John Jones, and Douglass Teschner, who each opened countless doors to me over the years. I am also exceedingly grateful to the colleagues and collaborators in Ukraine with whom I had the privilege of working and providing mutual support, including Tatiana Andreeva, Sergii Dvoryak, Konstantin Dumchev, Chuck Vitek, and my superlative research assistant, Hanna Dyatlenko.

I owe an enormous debt to Andriy Chybisov and Mika Bachmaha for their friendship and generosity. We three began our respective journeys into public health work in Ukraine in disparate places. After many years of collaboration in research and activism in Ukraine, chance and fate conspired to bring us together for a year in the same small neighborhood in Rhode Island. Nothing has challenged me, educated me, helped me innovate, or refined my thinking so much as the proximity we have been able to share in the past few years. How lucky I would be to continue working with you in the years to come.

Thank you to Gro and Pasha for making your home my home so many wonderful times. I love you both so dearly. Thank you to Heath, Inna, Yana, Hjordis, and Irina for your love and compassion—and for your willingness to, literally, walk into fire together. Thank you to Iryna, Scott, and Val for your eagerness to conspire and find ways to thwart restrictions on international funds transfers into Ukraine for the sake of our friends and loved ones. And thank you to the many individuals, whose names I cannot print here, who opened their doors, their work, and their lives to me throughout my research, who invested themselves in my education and awareness, and who trusted me to record their words and hear their stories. This book is the product of your labors and your trust in me. My greatest hope in all of this is that I have done you justice.

A Note on Language

Ukraine is, by and large, a bilingual country. The Russian and Ukrainian languages are both widely used, and most residents have at least a basic competency in both. As they are Slavic languages, Russian and Ukrainian share many words and grammatical forms; yet, they are distinct languages. Participants in my research chose to speak with me in Russian, Ukrainian, English, or even a mix of these, as was their preference. In this text, when words appear that are distinct to one language or the other, I mark them as such (e.g., Ukr: *zhittia*; Rus: *zhizn'*). When words appear that are homonyms and bear the same meaning in each language, I do not (e.g., *narkoman*). Many common first names have distinct Russian and Ukrainian forms. Though the names used in this text are pseudonyms, I have given monikers to participants that match their language of choice (e.g., *Sergey* vs. *Serhii*) and the level of formality we adopted in our conversations (e.g., *Dmitrii* vs. *Dima*). Readers familiar with these signifiers will be able to catch their meanings throughout the text, but those who are not familiar will not be missing very much. Place names in Ukraine also have distinct Russian and Ukrainian forms. In this text, I have chosen to use the Ukrainian form for all place names (e.g., Kyiv instead of Kiev), with the exception of the city of Odessa. The Ukrainian variant of Odessa contains only one "s"; however, the Russian form has become so standardized in English-language text that I chose to use this spelling variation instead. Odessa has, after all, earned the right to stand out a little bit.

A Glossary of Terms

anti-maidan: a loosely associated collection of social movements that were generally characterized by a pro-Russian or anti-European politics and organized in opposition to the EuroMaidan revolution and the political changes it triggered.

baiduzhist':   (Ukrainian) indifference.

bazhannia: (Ukrainian) desire.

Berkut: a special police force operated under the aegis of the Ukrainian Ministry of Internal Affairs, whose duties included the preservation of civil order within the sovereign territory of Ukraine. The Berkut was disbanded by an order of Ukrainian parliament in 2014.

Donbas: a region of eastern Ukraine that includes territories around the Donets'k River. Donbas is a shortening of Donets'k Basin.

EuroMaidan: a large antigovernment protest movement that originated in Kyiv in November 2013, but spread to many different cities in

Ukraine in the following months. The protests ended in the deaths of more than one hundred civilians due to police violence and the flight of President Viktor Yanukovych from Ukrainian territory.

gosudarstvo: (Russian) sovereign.

khoziaistvo: (Russian) domain.

narcology: a medical specialization recognized in Soviet medicine concerned with the prevention and treatment of "addictive" disorders.

narkoman: (Russian/Ukrainian) someone who uses drugs.

opiate: any pharmacological substance derived from opium, a latex excretion of the opium poppy. Codeine, morphine, and heroin (diacetylmorphine) are examples of natural opiates.

opioid: a term used to describe any pharmacological substance, whether natural or synthetic, which binds to opioid receptors in the brain. Methadone, fentanyl, and buprenorphine are examples of synthetic opioids.

ravnodushie: (Russian) indifference.

shirka: (Russian/Ukrainian) a slang term that refers to an opiate solution derived from poppy plants, which is commonly injected in Ukraine.

svoi: (Russian/Ukrainian) ours, our own.

zhelanie: (Russian) desire.

ABBREVIATIONS

AIDS   Acquired immune deficiency syndrome

DNR   Donets'k People's Republic (Rus: *Donetskaya Narodnaya Respublika*)

EU   European Union

HIV   Human immunodeficiency virus

LNR   Luhans'k People's Republic (Rus: *Luganskaya Narodnaya Respublika*)

MAT   Medication-assisted treatment

MoH   Ministry of Health

PEPFAR   President's Emergency Fund for AIDS Relief

SSR   Soviet Socialist Republic

WHO   World Health Organization

USAID   United States Agency for International Development

Map of Ukraine

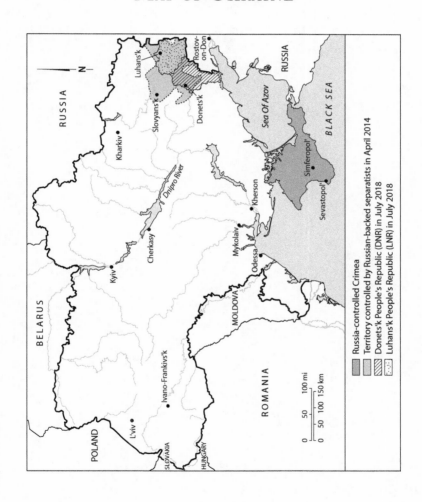

Russia-controlled Crimea

Territory controlled by Russian-backed separatists in April 2014

Donets'k People's Republic (DNR) in July 2018

Luhans'k People's Republic (LNR) in July 2018

Narkomania

INTRODUCTION

"Have you read Bulgakov?" This is a rhetorical question.

Elena and I stand side by side in a dusty clearing outside the methadone clinic's heavy gate.[1] Cars speed past us on the road to our right—a busy highway connecting the bedroom districts on the fringes of Kyiv City to the dense city center. I am waiting to meet someone. Elena has a cigarette and needs a light. We turn toward each other rather than squinting into the hot summer sun.

I have seen her at this clinic many times over the past few months. Her garish bleach-blonde hair and oversized sunglasses make her hard to miss. We have not been formally introduced, yet she has been an object of fascination to me for some time. She embodies an intense personality, prone to loud interruptions and exaggerated body movements. This rubs many of the other patients here the wrong way. Some, however, find virtue in her. I had seen her charged with child-care duties many times by fellow patients who, by choice or by circumstance, had come to the clinic with young ones in tow, choosing to let Elena fascinate them with games in the courtyard as their true guardians kept appointments with the clinic staff inside.

On this particular day, I find myself alone with Elena for the first time. To fill the silence I ask her what she thinks of the program. She responds with a question of her own: "Have you read Bulgakov?" After pausing to drag on her cigarette, she asks again. "*The Master and Margarita.* Have you read that one?"

Despite her low social status as a methadone patient and the pervasive stereotype that, as a consequence, she is poorly educated, immature, and stupid, Elena's expertise on classic Russian and Ukrainian literature is spectacular. Not only is she familiar with a broad canon of works, she can also quote long passages of fiction and poetry from memory, a true indicator of her *kul'turnost'*, her sophistication and fluency in the elements of "high culture." I, on the other hand, had never read anything by Mikhail Bulgakov, not even his most famous novel, *The Master and Margarita.*

Elena continued. "In that one, especially, he talks about the world in constant opposition, about everything being defined by good and bad, sacred and evil, black and white. And they must always arrive together, never alone. For me, I'd say it's pretty much like that."

Over time, I came to recognize Elena's assessment as typical: methadone therapy for the treatment of opioid use disorder was considered very good in some ways, but challenging in others. When I asked other patients how they liked being on methadone, most also structured their responses in terms of pros and cons—*plyusy* and *minusy*, as they are called in Russian and Ukrainian. The general consensus, though, was that this treatment option is ultimately a net positive for people struggling with opioid use disorder. One young man told me that joining this program had changed his whole life. There is, however, one significant *minus* to be taken into account: being in treatment doesn't necessarily change the social stigma that comes with the disease. When people look at you, I was often told, they don't see a patient; everyone still just sees an "addict."

I stand pondering Elena's words for a moment, lacking a witty comeback for sustaining our repartee. A dirt path stretches out in front of us and down across a dusty lawn that separates the clinic grounds from a large forest park. As it leads away, the path hooks around a small reservoir, which creates a bit of stillness between the traffic on either side. A sudden rustling of leaves from the tall reeds by the water catches our attention. A man emerges. Clean jeans.

Graying hair. I recognize him. He waves Elena over. She jolts to attention, drops her cigarette, and gallops off in his direction. "Don't leave!" she hollers back at me, "I'm not saying goodbye!" and then disappears with her husband into a secluded spot where no one can see them get high.

Elena was hard to pin down. She was an experienced user of opioids and other illegal substances and, therefore (as the stereotype goes), a low-class, no-good person. Yet she was extremely knowledgeable about art and literature and, therefore (as a different stereotype goes) a very high-class, respectable individual. She has been a regular patient at this methadone clinic for several years, never missing a day of her treatment. This makes her, on the one hand, an obedient, adherent, "deserving" patient (Parsons 1951). On the other, she also engages in different forms of drug use—perhaps nonopioid, but illicit nonetheless—in the context of certain social and familial relationships, potentially tarnishing her image, bringing into question how "worthy" a patient she really is. And, as her fellow patients illustrated, it was just as easy to love her as despise her—she provided ample fodder with which to justify either position. Elena can, and does, represent many different things to many different people.

This book is full of stories about people like Elena: about those who use illicit drugs, those in treatment, those out of treatment, and the various social worlds they occupy. More than this, though, this book is about the meanings that Elena and others like her bear for the powerful institutions that frame the world around them. It is about how these meanings are entangled in broader discourses of power and sovereignty; how these meanings are mobilized in efforts to construct national identity; how the geopolitical elite subject those like Elena to selective policing, rights violations, and other delimited forms of citizenship in an effort to consolidate power. Above all, this book is about the ways in which the marginalization of drug-using citizens has become a pervasive tool of statecraft both in and around Ukraine, and about how the manipulation of medical discourse around drug use can buoy up national identities, forging threads of continuity in times of rapid social and political change.

The patients receiving methadone at Elena's clinic are among the approximately eight thousand people in Ukraine receiving medication-assisted treatment (MAT) with pharmaceutical interventions like methadone (UNAIDS 2016). The goal of MAT is to help those with opioid use disorder regain control over their physical dependency to opioids through a

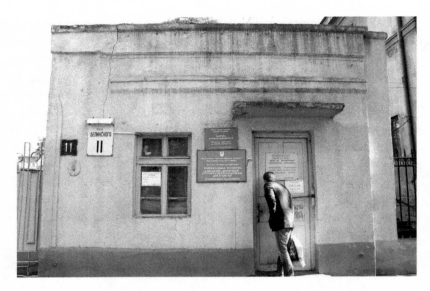

The entryway to a local hospital that provides MAT services. Photo by author.

strict regimen of prescription medications that stabilize their cycles of euphoria and withdrawal. Opioid agonist drugs used for MAT, specifically methadone and buprenorphine, help curb cravings for illicit opioids by binding to μ-opioid receptors in the brain, the same receptors that all opioids, including morphine and heroin (diacetylmorphine), bind to, thereby controlling withdrawal symptoms and cravings to use (Kosten and George 2002). The logic of this therapy is not unlike that of nicotine patches designed to help cigarette smokers quit smoking. It allows individuals to closely regulate and control their intake of a class of substances for which they have developed a physical dependence and alter the social milieu in which that consumption takes place. It provides the stability many need in order to address the larger issues that led to problematic substance use in the first place.

Ukrainians who use drugs exist at the epicenter of an internationally recognized public health crisis. Though they represent less than 1 percent of the total Ukrainian population (Bojko et al. 2015), they carry the lion's share of the country's HIV burden. Today, nearly one in five people who use drugs in Ukraine is living with HIV (UNAIDS 2015). Consequently, the HIV and opioid epidemics in Ukraine are practically synonymous in the public imagination. Groups like the United States Agency for International Development

(USAID), the U.S. President's Emergency Plan for AIDS Relief (PEPFAR), and the Global Fund to Fight AIDS, Tuberculosis, and Malaria (the Global Fund) have spent enormous amounts of money in support of MAT and other public health interventions designed to slow the spread of HIV in Ukraine and elsewhere. In 2016, the Ukrainian government pledged to financially support all MAT services in the country (UNAIDS 2016). Those promises translated into expenditures of nearly UAH 13 million (about USD 500,000) in the 2017 fiscal year (U.S. President's Emergency Plan for AIDS Relief 2018). At the time of my research (2007–14), all MAT programs in Ukraine were funded solely by international organizations.

By considering the trajectory taken by people who use drugs as they pass in and out of the various institutions that receive them, this book draws attention to how international public health campaigns create spaces rife with competing views of what "addiction" is, what MAT does, and what recovery from substance use disorder actually looks like. Many anthropologists have argued that biomedically oriented definitions of "addiction" often overlook the social factors that shape the patterns and meanings of drug use (Bourgois 2003; Garriott 2011; Meyers 2013; Spradley 1968). That disconnect between the biological and the social can, in turn, weaken the ability of biomedical interventions like MAT to adapt to patients' lived realities in different cultural contexts. Much ethnographic research on treatment for substance use disorders in the United States has also argued that biomedical frames tend to obscure the fact that many interventions for "addiction" are disciplinary technologies, and the forms that discipline takes can vary greatly across cultural divides (Bourgois 2000; Campbell 2007; Carr 2010; Meyers 2013). This observation holds true across diverse contexts, including Ukraine, because biomedical interventions do not simply act upon the body; they also act upon the body politic, the state-sponsored effort to ensure "the regulation, surveillance, and control of bodies (individual and collective) in reproduction and sexuality, in work and in leisure, in sickness and other forms of deviance and human difference" (Scheper-Hughes and Lock 1987, 7–8). Put another way, the rigidness of MAT's biomedical logic makes it useful for rendering people who use drugs "manageable" in a social sense in addition to keeping them "healthy" in a physical or biological sense (Bourgois 2000; Carr 2010; Foucault 1977).

The question of how or why people who use illicit drugs need to be managed, on the other hand, varies according to dominant ideological and cultural values. In the post-Soviet space, histories of war, language politics, planned economies, authoritative rule, and shared cultural experiences have generated theories of personhood, governance, and agency that are, in some ways, unique to this time and place. Caught in more than a simple opposition between seemingly "Western" notions of individualism and seemingly "Soviet" ideologies of collective society, Ukrainians today move through a kaleidoscope of political structures, social networks, and systems of reciprocity as they go about their daily lives. As medical anthropologist Michelle Parsons has observed, "Western social theorists often assume structure binds agency, while the [Eastern European] point of view is diametrically opposed: structure creates agency" (2014, 21). Informal practices of gifting, collaboration, bribery, innovation, and protectionism allow ordinary citizens to "make do" (Caldwell 2004) in a challenged, post-transition economy and supports "a strong ethos of collective responsibility, shared experience, and mutual assistance [that] continues to shape social life" (Phillips 2010, 239). What precisely is it, then, in this specific social and historical terrain, that Ukrainian physicians, politicians, and people who use drugs hope that MAT will manage? In the current zeitgeist of Eastern Europe's post-Soviet states, what personal, relational, or social ills does MAT seem poised to repair? And what are the implications for these essential public health services when shifts in sovereign power alter the answers to these questions?

How We Know What We Know about "Addiction"

Historian Mariana Valverde has argued that the dominant European view of "addiction" throughout the twentieth century understood this condition to stem from a deficiency—or, in Valverde's words, a "palsy"—of the will (1998). As the century progressed, many so-called addictive behaviors have become reclassified as disorders of the biomedical kind due to concerted efforts to draw alcoholism into the realm of biomedical authority and render it "a respectable disease" defined as "a malfunction of the individual, be it at the chemical, genetic, biological or psychological level" (Singer and Baer 1995, 303–4). However, as historian Nancy Campbell has observed, "[various] scientific efforts to explicate addiction have each answered [pertinent] questions differently, and . . . none have stabilized any one set of answers for long" (2007, 2). Those answers, in other words, have consistently proved confounding and slippery, and that very slipperiness seems to be a fundamental characteristic of the concept of "addiction" itself. In popular understanding, ideas about substance use and substance use disorders play on notions of physical health, mental health, social integration, desire, will, control, and identity, to name a few. As medical anthropologist Todd Meyers has observed, "addiction" does not "lend itself to straightforward ways of *knowing*" (2013, 20).

Consider, for example, how Nora Volkow, director of the National Institute on Drug Abuse at the U.S. National Institutes of Health (NIH) since 2003, has characterized "addiction" in her public remarks. In a 2006 presentation to the NIH's Clinical Center Grand Rounds, she described "addiction" as a disease of "disrupted volition" incurred through changes in dopamine levels in the nucleus accumbens of the brain (Volkow 2006). Nearly a decade later, Dr. Volkow delivered the convocation lecture at the Annual Meeting of the American Psychiatric Association, in which she presented a more refined explanation of this idea—yet one in which the biological and the philosophical were no less entangled: "[We] in psychiatry embrace addiction as a chronic disease of the brain, where the pathology is the disruption of the areas of the circuits that [enable] us to exert free will. That [enable] us to exert free determinations. Drugs disrupt these circuits" (Volkow 2015). As a highly respected scientist with considerable intellectual and scholarly prowess, Volkow nevertheless describes the action of these quantifiable brain activities through metaphor—through the fundamentally Western concept of "free will." Though cutting-edge technologies like neuroimaging have allowed scientists to pinpoint areas of the brain implicated in a variety of neurological pathologies or disorders—a technique of producing knowledge through the refutation of the immaterial, which Judith Butler has called "recourse to materiality" (2007, 165)—the questions of what consciousness, self-awareness, or free will are or are made of remain quite unsettled.

Even as the disease model of "addiction" has grown in evidence and momentum, Americans who lack the scientific training or professional motivation to engage with concepts like dopamine regulation and the functional role of the nucleus accumbens continue to find sufficient fodder for creating, communicating, and utilizing ideas about "addiction" through the moral values contained in these metaphors. Medical anthropologist William Garriott has considered the social impacts of "addiction" as a metaphor, arguing that "narcotics [are] a robust medium through which broader anxieties over immigration, poverty, and intergenerational conflicts, to name a few, are articulated by both citizens and the state" (2011, 6). In other words, it is not only possible but, indeed, relatively ordinary for us to engage the metaphor of free will to understand "addiction" in order to, in turn, use "addiction" itself as a metaphor for the social and ideological threats that society may face.

The longevity of this view in popular culture is important, given predictions that the medicalization of "addiction"—developed and adopted by numerous researchers throughout the twentieth century—would free individuals from the moral implications of their substance use disorder by reframing the condition as a disease, not a choice. Yet a quick scan of headlines regarding substance use in the United States will reveal that this fate has not entirely come to pass. Insofar as the un-moralization of illness states can be considered a function of medicalization, it would be appropriate to brand "addiction" as a disease that has always been never quite medicalized, thanks in large part to the ways in which elements of free will have been actively built into the clinical science of "addiction" for decades. Nancy Campbell has illustrated this fact well in her book *Discovering Addiction* (2007), in which she describes the main hubs of American substance use research in the mid-twentieth century: two clinical research institutes housed in all-male federal prisons—one in Lexington, Kentucky, the other in Fort Worth, Texas—nicknamed "The Narcotics Farms"—and a monkey colony maintained for controlled trials and narcotics testing at the University of Michigan. A key technological component of these trials was providing the monkeys, drugged with narcotics until physically dependent, with the ability to self-administer more narcotics. Lead researcher Maurice Seevers and his team used the animals' artificially produced capacity to self-administer drugs to draw connections between the animal behavior observed in his lab and human notions of preference or "liking." They argued that the monkeys' behavior amounted to "mimic[king] human self-medication and drug seeking" behaviors (Campbell 2007, 51). The idea that monkeys' willingness to administer drugs to themselves to the point of self-harm provided concrete justification for the definition of "addiction" as the drug-induced crippling of free will.

Qualitative research on substance use had been carried out since before these laboratory studies began. Bingham Dai, a sociologist at the University of Chicago, published a landmark study in 1937 that drew connections between the "maladjusted personality" or "general social disorganization" (Dai 1937) of the substance-using individuals he studied and Emile Durkheim's insights on social cohesion and anomie (Durkheim 1979). Ten years later, Alfred Lindesmith, also a University of Chicago sociologist, published a similar tome titled *Opiate Addiction* (Lindesmith 1947), in which he concluded that the development of addictive disorders rested on the patients' recognition of their withdrawal symptoms as related to the pain-relieving narcotic they had been receiving. Sociologist Howard Becker continued this legacy into the 1950s with studies of marijuana smokers and other so-called "social deviants." Yet, even in these decades, the social study of drug use seemed more of an oddity to most scholars than a growing field of research. As Becker later recalled, "no one was much interested" in what he and his predecessors had been doing (Becker 2015).

The contemporary ethnography of drug use did not emerge in full force until the 1990s, when "the revelation that 'certain risk groups,' including people who use heroin, had developed an immune disorder variously called GRID or AIDS (among other names) eventually led to the conclusion that any effort to understand and arrest the spread of this malady would need more drug ethnographers than were currently available" (Page and Singer 2010, 71–72). This period bore witness to major works on the sociocultural drivers of substance use, such as Philippe Bourgois's book, *In Search of Respect* (2003), in which Bourgois takes great pains to locate his informants' impetus to use and sell drugs in their exclusion from the primary economic market and, by extension, from legal means of earning a living.

In recent years, new and innovative approaches to substance use ethnography have emerged in answer to (or in rejection of) the fundamentally structural approach that defined the early research of Bourgois and his contemporaries on this topic. Maria Yellow Horse Brave Heart (2003) has proposed Historical Trauma theory, which illuminates historical and intrafamilial patterns that perpetuate high rates of alcoholism among Lakota families in North America. In a similar theoretical move, Angela Garcia (2010) has taken up the concept of melancholia, an idea originally developed by Freud, to explain frequent and occasionally violent recidivism among drug treatment patients in rural New Mexico. She contextualizes these behaviors within lengthy histories of material loss, personal dislocation, and social disenfranchisement. Todd Meyers's (2013) ethnography of adolescents in drug treatment in Baltimore explores the social and interpersonal effects that pharmaceutical intervention is expected to render. He scrutinizes the spaces "where the *clinical* and the *social* become difficult to distinguish" (Meyers 2013, 7). Equally compelling is E. Summerson Carr's (2010) description of the semiotic work undertaken by staff at American drug treatment centers for the purpose of imparting specific ideologies of relatedness and self-presentation to patients.

Each of these ethnographic efforts seeks to reveal something new about the social production of "addiction" and addicted bodies. Their purpose, writ large, is not to dispense with earlier theoretical modes, but to escape the reification of hegemonic concepts of "addiction" and the characterization of drug use as a visible, maladaptive, socially deviant behavior. They are, in a way, experiments in representation. They attempt to articulate substance use behaviors in terms of universally human qualities and shared modes of life, to reject the cultural logic that appeals to the socially marginalized state of drug use to justify the continued marginalization of these behaviors and the people who engage in them.

In this text, I build on the insights of these new literatures by considering not only how illicit drugs become tools for articulating (or, in some cases, coping with) social anxieties, but also how the social imagination of individuals who consume substances become the raw material for other kinds of social, ideological, or symbolic work. Further, I consider not only how the personal histories of Ukrainians who use drugs have shaped the experience of substance use in the context of their own trauma and dispossession but also how different chronologies and lived experiences produce shared understandings of "addiction" in a space steeped in legacies of socialism and social collectivization. Carr's ethnography of substance use treatment in the United States "illustrates the co-constitution of ideologies of language and personhood" and "that institutions [like substance use treatment programs] are organized by representational economies" (Carr 2010, 224). I consider how these representative "addiction imaginaries" shape not just individual subjectivities but the identity of entire nations.

Global Public Health in Ukraine

Driven by the shared mission of bringing contemporary medical technologies to low-resource regions of the world, international global health organizations often seek to relocate technologies developed in wealthy countries—frequently North America or Western Europe—into nations experiencing vastly different social and financial realities. Contemporary approaches to MAT that donors sought to implement widely in Ukraine, for instance, emerged out of North American biomedical logics about the neurobiology—and morality—of "addiction." In contrast, the medical science of "addiction" in the former Soviet sphere was founded upon a much more Cartesian, materialist view of human behavior. Soviet medical scientists understood problematic drug use to be driven by rigid neural pathways that developed over time as a result of repeated external stimuli and pathological behavior in response to those stimuli. Undoing those neural pathways, according to the founder of this approach, Dr. Ivan Pavlov, required long periods of time in therapeutic environments designed to provide contradictory stimulus and "re-wire" the "addicted" brain (Chilingaryan 1999). In this school of thought, maintaining opioid-dependent patients on opioid medications (like MAT) was viewed as a particularly self-defeating enterprise.

The use of methadone as a long-term treatment for opioid use disorder was first promoted by American clinicians treating heroin-dependent patients in the 1960s, at a time when heroin-related mortality was the leading cause of death for adults between fifteen and thirty-five years of age in New York City (Joseph and Appel 1993, 14). Most federal authorities on drug use in the United States, including the National Institute of Mental Health and the Drug Enforcement Agency, were against this approach throughout the 1960s and 1970s, due largely to the perceived dilemma of prescribing more opioids to people who were already opioid dependent (Joseph and Appel 1993, 14). As a result, federal regulations governing MAT were extremely restrictive until the emergence of HIV/AIDS in the 1980s. This new epidemic quickly prompted a change in U.S. and European public health priorities, helping MAT garner the reputation it still holds today as an essential and life-saving tool in the fight against HIV.

MAT is now included in the comprehensive package of services recommended by the World Health Organization (WHO) for combating HIV/AIDS worldwide, and methadone and buprenorphine, the two synthetic opioids used in MAT, are both on the WHO list of essential medicines (WHO 2010). Powerful international health organizations, like the Global Fund, have promoted and funded MAT in resource-limited settings around the world within the framework of a broad package of HIV control strategies. The Global Fund is arguably the most significant financial backer of MAT in low-income countries. This international group was founded in 2002 for the specific purpose of reducing the global burden of infectious diseases

(Global Fund 2016a). Worldwide, the Global Fund has disbursed more than USD 42 billion between 2002 and 2016, more than 75 percent of which it received from ten primary donor states: the United States, France, the United Kingdom, Germany, Japan, the European Union, Canada, Italy, Sweden, and the Netherlands (Global Fund 2016b).

Anthropologists working across resource-poor regions of the world have often critiqued global health efforts—like those supported by the Global Fund—as veiled attempts to cultivate ideal, governable subjects through the application of selective regulatory pressure (Dunn 2008; Keshavjee 2014; Koch 2013; Nguyen 2010). In this literature, "addicts," AIDS sufferers, and other "losers" of neoliberalism have been defined almost exclusively as the messy, tragic accidents of contemporary socioeconomic structures. This book offers a counterpoint to these claims, suggesting that marginalized, "throw-away" members of society may in fact be essential to the social fabric of the nation-state. Specifically, I argue that biomedically defined groups of social "Others" may be just as constitutive of contemporary social order as is the institutional pressure that produces neoliberal, or "self-governing," subjects. In this view, global health programs are about more than just human rights, and the medical and legal containment of people who use drugs entails not simply technologies of regulation and control. As the case of MAT in contemporary Ukraine makes clear, the success or failure of global health efforts (especially those directed toward social "Others") can also serve to validate national and cultural identity by bracketing an imagined population as the undesirable or undeserving "Other" of that identity.

Ukraine's Drug-Driven Epidemic

Ukraine's HIV epidemic came late, relatively speaking. Though the first recorded case of HIV in the Ukrainian Soviet Socialist Republic (SSR) was identified in 1987, the impact of the virus on public health in the region remained meager for the better part of a decade. In 1996, the rate of new HIV infection suddenly spiked among the social networks of Ukrainians who injected drugs, increasing the annual incidence of new infections from the low dozens into the thousands within a year's time (Hamers et al. 1997). According to Ukrainian social scientist Viktoriya Zhukova, state recognition of the significant HIV burden among people who inject drugs did little to help forestall the epidemic; rather, it "naturalized the IDUs [injection drug users] equals HIV formula by admitting that HIV was already there and refusing to dwell further upon the reasons which led to the increase in drug abuse in the newly independent state" (2013, 29). In other words, the social and political imaginaries that people who use drugs were sorted into as they entered into public awareness in Ukraine helped solidify noncritical thinking about drug use and its public health consequences as "common sense." Public and political discourse did not pursue the question of *why* HIV rates among people who inject drugs were so high.

Meager harm reduction efforts began popping up in major cities across Ukraine on the heels of this drug use-driven HIV epidemic. Local nongovernmental organizations (NGOs), occasionally powered by small donations from foreign charities and often led by individuals who had attained foreign university degrees, began distributing condoms, establishing syringe access programs, and launching social marketing campaigns to raise awareness about HIV. In Odessa, for example, a small organization named "Faith, Hope, and Love" began providing condoms and syringes to people who inject drugs in 1996 with the support of a USD 50,000 grant from the United Nations Children's Fund (UNICEF) (Foley 1998). In 1995 the Pasteur Institute funded a similar harm reduction effort in Simferopol, the administrative center of Crimea (Zalati, Iatsiuk, and Nepomniashchaia 2000). UNAIDS provided programmatic support to a syringe access program that opened in the northeastern city of Kharkiv in 1997 (Belyĭ 2000). Similar grassroots programs emerged around the same time in other regional centers, such as Mykolaiv (Hyde 1999), Vinnitsya (Polonets and Andrushchak 2000), and Cherkasy (Mitskaniuk 2000). Though these small efforts did attract some international attention, it was not until 2002 that Ukraine became meaningfully integrated into the international global health project of fighting HIV. That year, the Global Fund was formally created and began accepting applications from eligible nations to fund HIV prevention and treatment efforts. Ukraine's Ministry of Health (MoH) applied for funds and was successfully awarded a grant of USD 91 million, two-thirds of which was designated for HIV treatment and care (WHO 2005).

In the years immediately following the Global Fund's first financial commitment to Ukraine, things did not go quite as planned. Disagreements swelled between the Ukrainian government and its financial benefactor over spending priorities, health-care policies, and the role that civil society should play in public health efforts. Though ostensibly related to practical issues, these conflicts also stemmed from ideological differences about the nature of substance use and of HIV, differences fueled by the relative positions held by Ukraine and its donors in the international power structure. To begin with, independent Ukraine did not make much sense within the global landscape of HIV in the early 2000s. Recipients of international aid were typically developing nations located in the "Global South"—a region often defined in the Western imagination by weak health-care systems, financial precariousness, and populations of color. By these standards, Ukraine more closely resembled those wealthy nations pouring money into the Global Fund's coffers: the United States, France, Sweden, Germany, Canada, and the Netherlands, among others (Global Fund 2016b). Though it faced many challenges following the collapse of the Soviet Union, Ukraine was then and is now a low- to middle-income, predominantly white, European country with a high-functioning health-care system and a well-developed, professionalized medical sphere. Ukrainian society thus stands in stark contrast to the commonly held Western fantasy that global health work should "involve some combination of living with no running water/electricity, an outhouse, maybe a mud hut, hand washing clothes, and cooking over open fires" (Szabo 2011). For those doe-eyed humanitarians seeking such dire accommodations, Ukraine, with its luxury shopping malls, renowned symphony orchestras, and ubiquitous McDonald's franchises, is sure to disappoint.

Ukrainian leaders charged with the management of Ukraine's first HIV-prevention grant similarly failed to meet the Global Fund's expectations for its awardees. Through its philosophy of "country ownership" (Collins and Beyrer 2013), the Global Fund prioritizes the involvement of nonstate actors in national decision making. The promotion of this strategy often resulted in scenarios that irked the Ukrainian government, such as the Global Fund choosing to give financial support to nongovernmental organizations to hire social workers rather than granting the government those funds to expand the state health-care system. State actors complained that such policies undermined the sovereignty of the Ukrainian state, limiting its ability to set its own priorities (Zhukova 2013). As they were in possession of a complex and fully established state health-care infrastructure, founded upon nearly a century of Soviet institutional and political legacy, the Ukrainian government considered it unfit to capitulate to the pressures of a foreign entity seeking to reorganize the distribution of power.

By 2004, disagreement between the Ukrainian government and the Global Fund reached a breaking point. According to some reports, the final straw was the MoH's refusal to purchase antiretroviral medications through UNICEF, as the Global Fund had instructed. The MoH chose instead to spend their grant money through another company providing the same drugs at a cheaper rate (Berdychevskaya 2004; cited in Zhukova 2013). Also significant was the fact that the MoH was not disbursing the funds it was given for other purposes at all. Though Ukraine was expecting millions of dollars in payments from the Global Fund, the MoH only spent about USD 740,000 of the funds it was given during the first two years of its award (Parfitt 2004). At the time of my research, conventional wisdom among Ukraine's harm reduction advocates was that ministry officials delayed spending these funds because they could not find a way to evade the Global Fund's monitoring and embezzle a portion of the cash as it left the treasury. For all these reasons, the Global Fund announced in January 2004 that it was suspending its grant to Ukraine until such time as the money could be "redirected to a reliable organization" (Parfitt 2004).

In March 2004, the Global Fund selected the International HIV/AIDS Alliance in Ukraine (the Alliance), a Kyiv-based nonprofit that had only been operating independently from its Danish parent organization since the previous year, to serve as their primary grant recipient in Ukraine. The significant responsibility of managing a grant worth USD 15 million was transferred to this modest NGO for what was to be a trial period of one year (Bonn 2004). The organization responded admirably, expanding its staff and bringing on talented young professionals with public health training from prestigious foreign universities. As a result, the Alliance has remained the primary recipient of Global Fund monies for HIV prevention in Ukraine for many years. In December 2010, more than USD 300 million was pledged to Ukraine through the Global Fund's Round 10—one of the largest grants the Global Fund has ever offered; the Alliance was the primary recipient (U.S. President's Emergency Plan for AIDS Relief 2013).

Drug Use and the New Statecraft in the Post-Soviet Space

In 2005, medical anthropologist Michele Rivkin-Fish observed that ethnographers—with the exception of Adriana Petryna, whose work focused on the Chernobyl disaster (Petryna 2002)—had not yet "connected socioeco-nomic processes of disintegration and change after socialism with the chang-ing meanings of health, disease, and healing" (Rivkin-Fish 2005, 19). Since that time, medical anthropologists have enthusiastically filled that theoreti-cal void, bringing social subjectivities to bear on clinically relevant topics like infectious disease control (Koch 2013), mortality (Parsons 2014), medical pro-fessionalization (Bazylevych 2010), disability and welfare (Rasell 2013), HIV prevention (Owczarzak 2009), and TB care (Stillo 2015). Recent works have also explored Eastern European culture through the lenses of mental health care (Yankovskyy 2016), alcoholism (Raikhel 2016), substance use treatment (Lovell 2013; Zigon 2010), and self-determination (Matza 2014). These dis-cussions of health and health care are essential for understanding the tex-ture of subjectivity in postsocialist spaces, as the health of the human body serves as a potent metaphor for the "health" of society. To borrow a phrase from Carolyn Humphrey, "Metaphors express something important about how people are thinking about the changing social world around them. . . . This cannot but affect what happens in the future, since the ongoing repro-duction of a relationship or an organization is influenced by what people *think it is*" (2002, xxii).

In this book, I pursue an exploration of the "addiction imaginary" as a social metaphor in light of a question put forth by Petryna and Follis in their work on contemporary discourses of citizenship and human rights. "How," they ask, "are the limits of citizenship being probed along different lines, and what are the alternative pathways through which the political is being mo-bilized and through which citizens appear?" (2015, 402). This question brings to mind a similar one posed by Giorgio Agamben two decades earlier: "Where, in the body of [sovereign] power, is the zone of indistinction (or, at least, the point of intersection) at which techniques of individualization and totalizing procedures converge?" (1998, 6). In response to both of these, I ar-gue that the choice made by Ukraine's various sovereign bodies to enable or prohibit the functioning of MAT—as one of international global health's cor-rective "para-infrastructures" (Biehl 2013)—is able to forge or to sever a sig-nificant point of contact between the political and the biological, between the individual endowed with a "right to health" and the sovereign body that oversees the consummation and fulfillment of that right. More than simply a practical tool of governance wielded under the purview of the sovereign, such acts of selective inclusion and exclusion may also be constitutive of that very sovereignty—a tool of statecraft able to settle much of what becomes unsettled following rapid social and geopolitical change.

This pattern can be discerned in the political and military turmoil in which Ukraine has been embroiled since 2013. These conflicts have placed the "addiction imaginary" front and center in debates about the role of government and the limits of state entitlements. This has been especially true in exceptional or liminal spaces created by conflict, which can serve as "testing sites for the controlled expression of civil rights" (Ong 2006, 112). Aiwha Ong used this phrase to describe special autonomous regions in the People's Republic of China where foreign corporations can exploit a cheaper labor market without taking on the cost of tariffs associated with transporting their products into another sovereign state for processing. Within these spaces, governments can try their hand at constructing different, coeval forms of citizenship, building what Ong calls "'graduated' or 'variegated sovereignty'" (2006, 7). Similarly, three distinct zones of geopolitical crisis in Ukraine— the EuroMaidan protests in Kyiv, Russian-annexed Crimea, and the separatist-controlled territories in the eastern Donbas region—can also be viewed as experimental spaces where the relationships between citizenship, sovereignty, and citizens' entitlements are purposefully reconfigured. In each of these crises, the "addiction imaginary" has been an especially powerful foil against which claims of cultural unity or political legitimacy can be made.

The EuroMaidan protests, which began in Kyiv in November 2013, were a popular antigovernment movement that cohered around nominally democratic ideals about the role of the state and the entitlements of a free citizenry. These protests became known as "EuroMaidan," a portmanteau of the words "Europe" and "Maidan," a Ukrainian term for a city's central square. Following several acts of overt police violence against demonstrators, the protest camp in the city center quickly transformed into a paramilitary zone protected by elaborate defensive barricades built and overseen by the organization of Afghan War veterans with the aid of highly organized brigades of "self-defense" volunteers. Over the next several months, police violence on the outside of the square and more rigorous defensive organization on the inside of the square escalated in tandem until February 18–20, when a veritable war broke out between police and protestors, claiming the lives

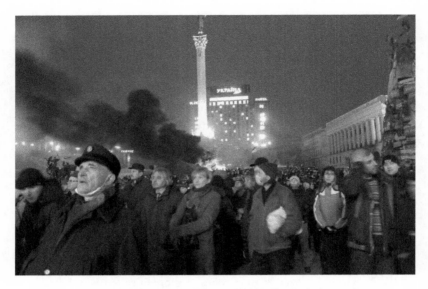

The EuroMaidan protest camp, February 20, 2014. Barricades burn to keep
the state police at bay after dozens of demonstrators were killed by police violence.
Photo by author.

of more than one hundred civilians. Lawyers, farmers, students, and even university professors were among the dead.

The "addiction imaginary" was pervasive in public discourse surrounding EuroMaidan. In particular, accusations of widespread substance use were frequently made by EuroMaidan protestors, EuroMaidan opponents, and other acting regimes in the region in order to discredit one another. On its face, the EuroMaidan protest camp was a socially and politically exceptional place believed by many to represent the sovereign Ukrainian nation in its purest form, unadulterated by the current government's corruption, greed, and loyalties to the Russian Federation. Tens of thousands of people were fed, clothed, provided with firewood and winter supplies, and offered free medical care including, when necessary, specialized treatment and trauma surgery. During the protests, activists felt and acted on a palpable urgency to ensure that all people were safe and cared for; however, this inclusive ideology was met by an equally powerful drive to exclude those who were deemed unworthy or dangerous, such as state actors, state police, and anti-Maidan protestors. Each of these groups was called dehumanizing names by those inside the

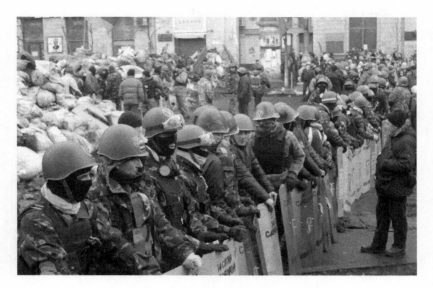

Self-defense groups man the barricades at EuroMaidan. Photo by author.

EuroMaidan camp: animals, zombies, prostitutes, and "addicts." Similar accusations of brainwashing, "addiction," or simply inducing a drug-addled psychological state, were hurled back at EuroMaidan protestors by opposing government actors and media outlets in both Ukraine and Russia. A favorite accusation of my own, which circulated in less-reputable social media forums, held that the massive barricades that EuroMaidan protestors had made of snow and ice were, in fact, constructed out of sandbags filled with drugs and that the water poured over them to create ice in Kyiv's subfreezing temperatures was, in fact, liter upon liter of vodka. Even the fighters on either side of the conflict, those who risked their lives over this disagreement about the future of Ukraine, could find common ground in the belief that people who use drugs were the enemy of a good society, however you define it.

The consequences of these events moved out of the realm of inflammatory rhetoric and into the practical world of public health policy when the Russian Federation subsequently took control of Ukraine's Crimean peninsula. On February 23, 2014, Ukrainian president Viktor Yanukovych succumbed to the pressures of the protest movement and fled in the night to

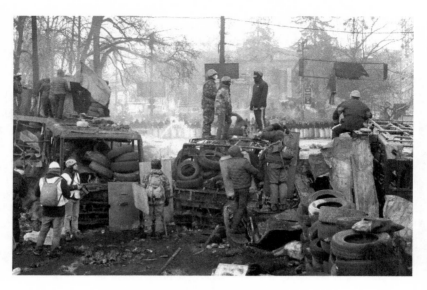

Defensive barricades at EuroMaidan. Photo by author.

the Russian town of Rostov-on-Don. In what appeared to be a direct response to Yanukovych's abdication of control, Russian soldiers quickly invaded the Autonomous Republic of Crimea and facilitated a military coup. New policies ushered in the dissolution of Ukrainian police and military establishments, the systematic oppression of ethnic minority Tatar communities living on the peninsula, and the reformation of the health-care system with the express purpose of disenfranchising Crimeans who use drugs. On April 2, 2014, Viktor Ivanov, then the head of the Russian Federation's Drug Control Service, publicly announced his intention to close all MAT programs in Crimea (Dunn and Bobick 2014), as MAT programs are illegal under Russian law. Ivanov characterized his desire to manage Crimeans who use drugs in eugenic terms, saying, "The 'rejuvenation' of drug addiction in recent years and the increasing number of female drug addicts [in Crimea] is causing a rise in the number of births of children with various disabilities, which is a threat to the gene pool" (Ivanov 2014). About eight hundred patients were receiving MAT in Crimea when the shutdown occurred, of which more than one hundred have since died due to overdose, suicide, and other fatal outcomes widely known to follow the abrupt cessation of treatment (Cornish et al. 2010; Davoli et al. 2007; Degenhardt et al. 2009).

As events in Crimea were unfolding, Ukrainian regions bordering the Russian Federation to the east and the Black Sea to the south experienced increasingly volatile protests against the post-EuroMaidan government of Ukraine. By the summer of 2014, local dissension in the Donets'k and Luhans'k regions received enough financial and military support from the Russian Federation to create an armed insurgency, sending this part of Ukraine into a violent separatist war that has raged for nearly four years, as of the time of writing. Territories claimed by fighters in these breakaway regions have been reorganized by local leaders (many of them veterans of Russian military and security forces) into semifunctioning autonomous zones dubbed the Luhans'k People's Republic (LNR) and the Donets'k People's Republic (DNR), respectively. The Ukrainian government has refused to acknowledge either the autonomy of these regions or the legitimacy of the separatist movement, designating the DNR and LNR as terrorist organizations (Chernichkin 2014). Nevertheless, separatist leaders have sought to establish a new sovereignty over the region distinct from the practices they view as characteristic of the Kyiv government. This military occupation has had predictably devastating effects on public-health programs, including MAT and HIV treatment. Furthermore, a significant element in the DNR leadership's agenda for bringing the separatist region "to order" was the focused persecution of those accused of drug using and drug dealing in the area and the meting out of violent punishments for their alleged social transgressions (Owczarzak, Karelin, and Phillips 2015).

In each of these conflict zones—the EuroMaidan protests, Russian-controlled Crimea, and the occupied eastern territories—the human rights of people who use drugs have shrunk to serve the needs of the politically powerful. As the dominant biopolitics shifted across these regions, the strategies used to manage the citizenry's individual and collective bodies, the very concept of citizens' "right to health," was retooled as well. Though Ukrainians who use drugs are not the only ones who have suffered under these transitions, they have nevertheless been used like chess pieces in these multiple attempts to assert (or reassert) new forms of social and political order. A close analysis of "the addiction imaginary" in these experimental political spaces reveals how current imaginations of sovereignty across this part of Eastern Europe collectively rest on the assumption that the enfranchised citizenry is a social collective (Collier 2011; Dunn 2008), one that the state is obliged to protect from the threat of dangerous, destructive, or exploitative "Others."

Creating sovereignty, therefore, requires an "Other" for the citizenry to be protected *against*, and people who use drugs have proved to be a popular and effective figment with which to fill that role.

An Ethnography of Exclusion

Though this is a book about public health, the arguments I make here are not based on incident rates or relative risk calculations. The subjects of my analyses are cultural values and systems of meaning, which require lengthy (and occasionally unstructured) engagement with ethnographic methods to capture and share. Ethnography can be defined as "the culmination of listening and observing and experiencing so many stories that they start to overlap, change, and repeat until the spectrum of responses have been collected and some agreement on general patterns and themes is established" (Chapman and Berggren 2005, 151). Participant observation, a key method of ethnographic research, likewise "unfolds in real time and captures the texture and rhythm of real life less mediated by researcher questions that shape and direct informant responses" (Chapman and Berggren 2005, 151). In practice, this can mean adopting new behaviors such as sharing cigarettes and cell phone minutes, standing in line at the bus depot together, assisting with child-care duties, and receiving instruction on fruit canning or backgammon strategy. As ethnographers, we develop long-term relationships with key informants and constantly foster what we hope to be genuine and mutual social connections.

My research is ethnographic in this most fundamental sense, defined by lengthy periods of residence in Ukraine and the cultivation of numerous personal and professional relationships during that time. Since 2007, I have been conducting observations in harm reduction agencies and MAT clinics, interviewing doctors, social activists, and people who use illicit drugs throughout central, southern, and western Ukraine. My longest stay lasted nearly a year and a half, stretching from the fall of 2012 to the spring of 2014, during which time I began systematically interviewing current and former MAT patients in several major urban centers. Throughout my research, I have also sought the support and expertise of public health experts—both Ukrainian and foreign—working on issues related to drug use and infectious disease in the region. Spending such long periods of time living in Ukraine has also afforded me opportunities to attend local harm reduction conferences, trainings hosted by Global Fund and USAID contractors to teach North American methods to Ukrainian social workers, and nationwide stakeholder meetings held in preparation for the tenth round of applications to the Global Fund.

Though my work has taken me to numerous regions of Ukraine to visit staff and patients at the few and widely scattered MAT programs in operation, I have spent longer periods of time, gaining a more intimate familiarity with local practices and routines, at MAT clinics in two major cities: Kyiv and L'viv. During the summer of 2013, I spent a great deal of time at a single methadone clinic in Kyiv's left bank bedroom communities. This clinic is where I met Elena. Staffed by two physicians, a social worker, and a steady rotation of nurses, it serves about 120 clients at any given time. I spent many long mornings in the courtyard of this clinic eating fresh cherries, watching backgammon games, and sharing the daily boredom with patients who found temporary respite in the patches of shade outside the entryway. Through these informal interactions, I bore witness to the evolution of social relationships and learned of the concerns that shaped these patients' daily lives. In addition to the general observations I made over several months, I conducted lengthy interviews with many of the medical staff and clients at this clinic.

In the fall of 2013, I spent several weeks shadowing clinicians and outreach workers in the city of L'viv and the surrounding rural areas. L'viv is a much smaller but culturally significant city in the west. Once part of Poland, the café-lined streets and pre–World War I architecture give L'viv a distinctly European—even bohemian—feel. This region is also home to strong nationalist sentiments and conservative social politics that place powerful taboos on topics like sex, abortion, racial integration, and, of course, substance use. While conducting my research there, I spent several weeks traveling around to various small towns in the L'vivska region with the staff of a local outreach organization that provided mobile syringe access services and rapid HIV testing. These services were offered out of a small, converted minibus, which carried a nurse and two social workers to scheduled stops around the region. Between twenty and fifty individuals received services from this mobile service point on any given day. When not accompanying these outreach workers on service runs, I spent time at a clinic that offered MAT near L'viv city center. The head physician at this clinic was fiercely dedicated to his work and was eager to speak to me about the needs of his patients and the many ways, physical and spiritual, in which he sought to help them. This clinic served about fifty patients in total. A number of individuals received services regularly from both this MAT clinic and the harm reduction outreach program.

Throughout most of my fieldwork, I worked independently, making decisions for myself about where to go, what to observe, and whom to interview according to the various matters I wished to explore. However, when the EuroMaidan revolution emerged in the winter of 2013, my relationships with key informants flip-flopped. Previously, I had reached out to them with requests for assistance when my needs arose. At the start of the revolution, a close contact from the L'vivska region began calling me to request that I accompany her and her friends to different protest events in Kyiv, where I was living. They would regularly drive in from L'viv to take part in the swelling political action. Some took months off of work to spend long stretches in Kyiv and support the protests. I spent a significant amount of time engaged in the public and private logistics of EuroMaidan with these contacts, who soon became very close and trusted friends. They offered themselves as constant and enthusiastic guides to the complex social structure of the protests. With their assistance, I was able to observe and record emerging events as they unfolded.

Though my permanent residency in Ukraine came to an end in the spring of 2014, my ethnographic work has not yet concluded. I was present in Kyiv during the forced annexation of Crimea that took place in February 2014, but was in the United States when, a month later, a military conflict germinated in the eastern regions of Donets'k and Luhans'k. I followed these events closely thanks to the frequent use of social media by Ukrainian soldiers fighting to regain control of these regions. I also knew personally a number of soldiers who volunteered to fight separatist forces in the east. Their regular updates and our frequent conversations online proved invaluable to my understanding of these events. Unfortunately, much less is known about the state of the individuals I met in Crimea. Very few people have been able to gain access to the peninsula since the annexation. Crossing the new border from mainland Ukraine is not easy, and many have been denied permission to do so on political grounds (Tomkiw 2016). The International HIV/AIDS Alliance in Ukraine has been able to maintain contact with and even trace the path of a few former MAT patients in Crimea as they scattered after the closure of their treatment programs. The violence experienced by some of these individuals is, therefore, known. For many others, however, the losses they have suffered can only be known indirectly.

Using this combination of firsthand ethnographic data and secondary data collected through multiple social and professional connections, this book follows the trajectory of people who use drugs through this array of institutions, events, and upheavals. I also trace the evocation of the "addiction imaginary" in these contested spaces to show how the exclusion of people who use drugs—whether they are people imagined or in the flesh—is a point of self-actualization around which so many declarations of personhood, citizenship, and sovereignty converge. What emerges from this analysis is a clear picture of how essential medicalized "Others" can be to the current sociopolitical order, forced to live in a state of exclusion that is demanded by the creation of the ideal body politic and those other, more "deserving" individuals under its banner.

Narkomania

The first half of this book explores the global response to HIV and the implementation of that response in Ukraine. Chapter 1 explores contemporary cultures of substance use in Ukraine and maps the social drivers that shape individual trajectories into substance use and, sometimes, into treatment. Chapter 2 describes the mechanisms of accountability that are used in Ukraine's HIV prevention efforts. It tells stories of statistical subterfuge collected from clinics across Ukraine to illustrate that relationships between the "local" and the "global" are dynamic and dialectical; that the boundaries between international standards of practice and clinic-based cultures are not always clear. Chapter 3 focuses more closely on the clinical spaces where medical providers and people who use drugs interact. It details how clinicians culturally construct people who use drugs as certain ideal types characterized by a certain affliction, as well as how those people, in turn, seek to define themselves against these clinical narratives. Both doctors and patients in MAT programs frequently cite desire as the most significant factor in determining the success of treatment: desire to be treated, desire to get better, desire to live. This emic view of substance dependence informs the social imagination of people who use drugs as weak-willed, partial citizens who cause problems for others but can't solve any of their own.

The second half of this book traces the social careers of people who use drugs outside the clinic, exploring the roles they play in popular imaginations of citizenship and government, which lie at the heart of the geopolitical conflict in this region. Chapter 4 contrasts two political performances: first, written correspondence between the Alliance and the Ukrainian MoH about MAT reform and, second, the public activities of a satirical political candidate who has adopted the persona of the *Star Wars* villain Darth Vader. Together, these sets of practices reveal the plasticity of the "addiction imaginary" in Ukraine and its utility for defining the sovereign state and the citizenry it serves. Chapter 5, through an analysis of the political discourses of EuroMaidan, considers the tenacity of the social marginalization experienced by people who use drugs. In this chapter, I argue that new forms of national sovereignty were enacted by EuroMaidan protestors through the construction of opposition members as "addicts" and through the metaphor that defines an "addict" as a spiritual slave. These generative discourses about citizenship and collectivity bring into sharp relief how clearly notions of civic personhood are defined in opposition to the negative stereotypes of wanton destructiveness often applied to people who use drugs. Finally, chapter 6 describes the practical and political consequences for people who use drugs of the separatist conflict in the east and the Russian annexation of Crimea. I argue that policy shifts under these new governments have served both as statements about what types of personhood are considered acceptable by governing powers and as demonstrations that the citizenship rights of undesirable subjects could, at any time, be revoked. In short, the new leaders of these regions purposefully reestablished state sovereignty by publicly excising part of the population framed as dangerous, fundamentally changing the bounds of their citizenry.

The main argument of this book is encapsulated in its title: *Narkomania*. It's Slavic cognate, *narkomaniia*, has two distinct and equally important meanings. First, this word, which carries the same meaning in Russian and Ukrainian, can be translated literally as "addiction." Derived from the Greek roots "narkō" (stupor) and "mania" (craze), this term signals the same uncontrolled obsession or excitement indicated by similar terms like "kleptomania" and "egomania." "Addiction" is a fundamentally cultural construct (Garriott and Raikhel 2015; Lindesmith 1968; MacAndrew and Edgerton 1969; Page and Singer 2010) capable of generating multiple understandings of who (or what) "addicts" are. Like "addiction," the Ukrainian concept of *narkomaniia* is also a social construct. It is distinct from the medical diagnosis of substance use disorder, a condition with a standard medical definition that can only be diagnosed through the appearance of key clinical symptoms, such as physiologically apparent withdrawal and increase in ability to control drug-consumption behaviors (WHO 1992).[2] In acknowledgment of this distinction, I use the terms "substance use disorder" or "opioid use disorder" to refer to these strictly defined clinical diagnoses. I use *narkomaniia*'s English equivalent, "addiction," to refer to the set of socially constructed ideas that constitute popular meanings of problematic substance use, its causes, its symptoms, and the forms of corrective action it is believed to require (Kleinman 1988).

The second meaning of the book's title, *Narkomania*, captures how such beliefs about people who use drugs are employed to articulate ideological norms about society at large. This occurs because culturally inflected views of "addiction," what I call the "addiction imaginary," can be mapped onto multiple constellations of moral and social anxieties. In Ukraine, as in much of Eastern Europe, the "addiction imaginary" gives breath to an ideology that discriminates between individuals according to their perceived mental freedom, according to their ability to be deliberate agents of their own free will. Nikolas Rose calls this an "ethopolitics," a system of ethics that "concerns itself with the self-techniques by which humans should judge and act upon themselves to make themselves better than they are" (Rose 2007, 27). Similar to the value that mainstream American culture places on individuality and self-reliance, Ukrainian culture holds up willfulness and sober self-determination as the ideal manifestation of the social self. To index these abstract social and moral constructs, I use the term *narkomaniia*, in lieu of "addiction" or its biomedical analogue, "substance use disorder," to underscore to broader ethopolitical discourses in Ukraine, which evoke a readily available "addiction imaginary" to help make sense of contemporary social and geopolitical realities.

This social *narkomaniia* is why neighbors accuse each other's children of drug use when conflict arises (see chapter 3). It is why Viktor Ivanov claimed that "participants in the Maidan riot were under the influence of drugs" (*Voice of Russia* 2014). It is why Russia inaugurated its rule over the annexed region of Crimea by shuttering MAT clinics and purposefully redrawing the boundaries of its citizenry, removing those who use drugs from the worthy populace (see chapter 6). It is why a young activist, dressed as Darth Vader, marched through the streets of Odessa with a phalanx of Storm Troopers, filming their violent raids of "drug dens" in the heart of the city (see chapter 4). Multiple configurations of the Ukrainian public can be seen, I argue, as possessed by *narkomaniia* in this sense, guided by a culturally contingent ethopolitics (Rose 2007) that facilitates the work of charting out shifts in social and political value through references to people who use drugs as toxic "Others." This book describes the cultural and political backdrop against which these events take place and explores how global health efforts supporting MAT in Ukraine allow these modes of thought to resonate more broadly into international politics and echo into the heart of the Ukrainian body politic.

Above all, I contend that evolving strategies for the medical and legal containment of people who use drugs in Ukraine must be viewed not simply as a matter of public health or human rights but as a potentially antihumanist tool of statecraft. In their efforts to establish what they perceive to be the ideal social order, the Global Fund, the Ukrainian government, EuroMaidan revolutionaries, the Russian Federation, and even separatist leaders in the Donbas region exploit people who use drugs. Ultimately, people who use drugs are useful for explaining contemporary conflicts, because the "addicted imaginary" is very useful to think with, and the social and structural violence frequently meted out against people who use drugs is nothing less than a demonstration of the state's ability to wield sovereign control over its own citizenry. In this way, the fulfillment or denial of their access to essential health technologies, such as MAT, can serve as a litmus test through which the question of sovereign authority can become settled in a politically contested space. In this postsocialist place, throttled by revolution and war, MAT programs and the people they serve become politicized, linking the availability or absence of care to the role of the state and the imagined society that will take shape tomorrow according to the moral order of today.

Chapter 1

HOMEGROWN

The Black Sea is an important part of this story. It will appear in this book again and again as a gateway or a barrier, as a moment of calm or a sign of sudden conflict. The Black Sea marks the beginning of the story I wish to tell. It is also where this story meets its end. At least, it is an end of some kind.

In 1774, Catherine the Great took control of the lands bordering the north shores of the Black Sea: territories that are, today, in southern Ukraine. Signing a peace treaty with the Ottoman Empire and marking the end of the Russo-Turkish war, she garnered sovereign authority over the seaports at Azov and Kerch, the Crimean Peninsula, and significant portions of land west of the Dnipro River. This expansion of tsarist control settled long-standing conflicts between Russians, Tatars, Poles, and Cossacks who all had vied for control over this fertile terrain for more than a century. Catherine thus recovered lands she felt had been previously "torn away" from her state, returning this region to what she and her contemporaries saw as its culturally and historically appropriate place within the Russian Empire. She named this region Novorossiia, the New Russia (Reid 1997).

The Black Sea port city of Odessa, mainland Ukraine's southernmost urban center, is a testament to Catherine's grandiosity as well as her expansionist tendencies. Built in 1794 to serve as the administrative seat of her new territories, Odessa quickly became a thriving center of culture and trade. Between 1819 and 1859, Odessa was a free port that attracted a diverse population of immigrants including Albanians, Armenians, Germans, Greeks, Romanians, Turks, and Poles. Odessa was also home to a large Jewish community, which grew to nearly 40 percent of the city's population by the end of the nineteenth century. In 1897, more than fifty different languages were spoken there (Richardson 2008). During World War I, Odessa was first occupied by the German army, only to be quickly reclaimed by Bolshevik forces that were pushing the borders of their new socialist state westward (Snyder 2012). The city was subsequently incorporated into a short-lived, independent state called the Ukrainian People's Republic, then reincorporated the following year into the even shorter-lived Odessan People's Republic, and then into the Ukrainian Soviet Socialist Republic (SSR), which came into being in 1919 (Plokhy 2017). Despite this rapid succession of occupations and statehoods, each harboring a new political agenda, the rich multiculturalism that had long defined Odessa persisted and survives to this day. This diversity affords Odessans a unique social identity that, in the local view, sets them apart from the rest of the region: they may be Ukrainian citizens, but many are Odessans, first and foremost.

In addition to its cultural and historical distinctions, Odessa is significant epidemiologically. It is where HIV first claimed a foothold in Ukraine. Though the virus appears to have emerged in the Ukrainian port cities of Odessa and Mykolaiv simultaneously (Nabatov et al. 2002), Odessa bore witness to the first major outbreak in 1996. During that year, the number of reported HIV cases rose from just a handful to nearly two thousand (Babenko 1996). The virus spread through Ukrainian social networks like wildfire, and rates of infection grew thirty-four-fold between 1995 and 1999 (Kobyshcha 1999). By 2016, an estimated 240,000 people in Ukraine were living with HIV, and an additional 38,000 had already died from AIDS-related diseases (UNAIDS 2018).

That this tidal wave of HIV infection was driven by injection drug use was then, and remains now, incontrovertible. Ukrainians who inject drugs constituted more than 70 percent of all known HIV cases in 1995 and as many as 80 percent of all known cases in 1998 (Kobyshcha 1999). The results of early epidemiological surveillance among people who use drugs drew a similarly bleak picture. As early as 1996, nearly one out of every five people who inject drugs in Odessa and nearly one out of every three in Mykolaiv were already living with HIV—truly staggering numbers by any standard (Hamers et al. 1997). Since that time, public opinion in Ukraine has saddled those living with HIV with personal responsibility for the disease (Carroll 2013, 2016a, 2016b; Mimiaga et al. 2010). The tragedy, according to the popular view, is not that people who inject drugs are acquiring HIV and dying of AIDS-related diseases; rather, the tragedy is that such morally debased people had turned up in Ukraine in the first place, many of them, it has been thought, hitting ground along the shores of the Black Sea—bursting through the thin, watery membrane that separated Ukraine from the rest of the world.

In Western public health discourse (in regions of North America and Europe, especially), substance use is very often associated with its individual health consequences: bacterial infections, viral diseases, overdose. In contrast, social scientists have historically viewed substance use of all kinds in cultural, rather than biomedical, terms. As early as the mid-twentieth century, sociologists from the University of Chicago, like Alfred Lindesmith and Howard Becker, were taking a social constructionist approach to substance use, arguing that people have to learn how to use, experience, and even enjoy drugs. Becker, for example, argued that someone smoking marijuana has to master three different skills before they are able to experience a real "high": (1) to learn to smoke, (2) to learn to recognize the effects of smoking, and (3) to learn to anticipate, talk about, and enjoy those effects with other people (Becker 1953). By the 1970s, anthropologists were applying methods of cognitive anthropology in their research, seeking to develop taxonomies of cultural categories and cognitive frames that shaped the experiences of people who use drugs. This approach often shed light on the effects of class divisions on the social acceptability of substance use. Anthropologist Mike Agar, for example, observed that "the implicit social environment against which behavior is measured as 'adaptive' or 'maladaptive' is that of the psychiatrist—white, upper-middle-class" (1973, 125), interpreting the so-called maladaptation of his research participants at the Lexington Kentucky Clinical Research Center as an artifact of a class culture that was not their own.

In this analysis, I combine these approaches to adopt a biocultural view of substance use, by which I mean that narcotic drugs have similar and predictable effects on the human body, but our lived experiences of those effects can be highly malleable. All opioids act as analgesics and as central nervous depressants, or sedatives, in the human body. These characteristics are, with some rare exceptions, invariable. Significant variation *does* exist, however, in the sociocultural and material environments in which those human-chemical interactions take place, and these local contexts shape so much more than how the effects of drugs feel to us when we take them. Economic forces, technological variation, social relationships, power differentials, market structures, and even gender norms influence practices of substance use, the interpretation of substance use experiences, and the meanings applied to those practices on a broader social scale.

In adopting this biocultural view, I follow a growing cohort of contemporary ethnographers who have forged new ways of thinking about substance use. I follow E. Summerson Carr, who sees "addiction treatment as a site where ideologies of language are refined and reproduced, processing people along the way" (2010, 233), by looking at how the way we talk about substance use informs the way we think about people who use drugs. By looking at the effects of larger social and governmental forces on substance-using bodies, I follow Philippe Bourgois, who describes marginalized classes of people who use drugs as "lumpen . . . a subjectivity that emerges among population groups upon whom the effects of biopower have become destructive" (Bourgois and Schonberg 2009, 19). In situating contemporary drug use in places like Odessa within the larger sociopolitical history of the region, I follow Angela Garcia, whose ethnography of heroin use in the Rio Grande valley highlights "how the historical and continuous process of dispossession of Hispano property and personhood emerge as a condition of possibility for the contemporary phenomenon of heroin use" (2010, 10). I follow Todd Meyers, who observed that "the evidence of ['addiction' treatment] success is not always the same between research and clinical practice, and between the various actors inside and outside the clinic the difference is even more pronounced" (2013, 7), by presenting a plurality of understandings about substance use and treatments for substance use disorder.

In sum, the biocultural view brings many facets of drug use in Ukraine into examination: language, history, systems of knowledge, the circulation of people and ideas both inside and beyond the walls of the clinic. Certain decisions about whether or not to use drugs, to initiate medication-assisted treatment (MAT), to accept certain risks, or to make strategic choices in the clinic or in life, can thus be seen in a new light, revealing familiar strategies for creating and defending a sense of self in a troubled social and chemical terrain.

Bricks and Mortar

The geography of health care for people who use drugs in Ukraine is constantly changing. This is due in part to the capricious nature of funding for harm reduction programs. This, along with the frequent couching of essential services in time-limited research or development projects, leads to the constant shuffling and reshuffling of services into different administrative schemes and physical spaces. When I traveled to Odessa in 2013, six years after my first visit there, I took a colleague who had been collaborating with MAT clinics in the area to visit the site of the city's first pilot methadone program, where I had spent time interviewing patients and staff in 2007 (see chapter 2). We walked for a few minutes into the city center until we came across a caged stairwell leading down to a basement apartment, the minor details of which I still remembered so well. My friend was astonished; he had been deeply involved in the improvement of MAT programs in Odessa for the better part of two years, but he had no idea that any such clinic had ever existed in that space. Though he was certainly the better expert on Ukraine's public health response to drug use, my historical awareness of this landscape outstripped his own by several years; ethnographic work can be funny like that.

This programmatic transience has another, deeper origin, however: the Soviet medical infrastructure of Ukraine, which has, for the most part, continued operating unchanged since the country gained independence in 1991. Major design decisions that informed the structure of the Soviet system long predated contemporary health concerns, like HIV and opioid use disorder. Consequently, health-care services for managing these diseases didn't necessarily have a natural "home" in the existing health care system. When the MoH of Ukraine established specialized HIV hospitals around the turn of the century, they housed these new facilities in a variety of hand-me-down buildings owned by the state. For example, one of the dedicated HIV hospitals in Kyiv—home to both an intensive care inpatient facility and an outpatient MAT program—boasted elaborate rococo-inspired embellishments on the

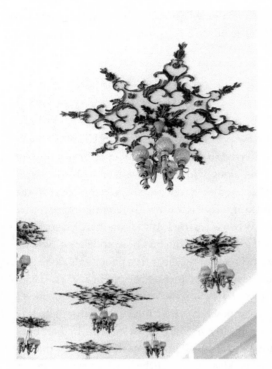

Decorative ceilings in a building now used as an HIV hospital in Kyiv. Photo by author.

walls and ceilings of one of its larger meeting rooms, betraying its past life as some kind of elite clubhouse or banquet hall.

When MAT began to expand beyond its first pilot sites in the late 2000s, some programs were able to situate themselves in spaces designated for narcological medicine—a Soviet medical specialization centered on the treatment and prevention of alcoholism and other "addictive" conditions. Despite their apparent similarities, narcology and MAT were a poor match for each other. The Soviet medical system was loosely founded on the belief that disease and illness were the products of social inequalities and exploitation experienced in the capitalist market (Field 1953), and the field of narcology, specifically, emerged in the mid-twentieth century at a time when alcohol-related mortality became perceived as a minor social problem (Lovell 2013). The goals of narcology, however, went beyond the clinical management of "addicted" bodies to include legal aspects of illicit narcotics use and the social aspects of substance use in the community. Medical anthropologist

Eugene Raikhel, who has conducted extensive research on alcohol use disorder in contemporary Russia, has observed that the work of narcologists, even today, is "authorized as much by the legal provisions for compulsory treatment and the intermeshing of medical and juridical organizations in the Soviet narcological service as by their medical credentials" (2016, 10). Anthropologist Anne Lovell has gone further, describing narcology as a field that "depict[s] patients under the influence of narcotics as lacking self-control and awareness of the danger they pose to self and society or the state. This problem of social volition was the justification for necessary incarceration—either forced hospitalization or prison" (2013, 139). MAT, as an individualized, outpatient, pharmacological treatment, is an anomaly in the world of narcology, which would classify the use of medications like buprenorphine and methadone as the pointless substitute of one narcotic for another. And yet, even as some narcologists in Ukraine remained firmly opposed to MAT, others proved to be some of its most dedicated advocates.

The MAT program where I met Elena (see the Introduction) was led by one such narcologist, who sought to make a comfortable space in difficult settings. The program was housed in a long-standing narcological clinic on the outskirts of Kyiv's left-bank sleeping districts. Compared to the banquet hall-turned-HIV hospital on the other side of town, this dispensary was a humble affair: a single-story cement building that sat along a busy highway, tucked just out of sight behind a strategically placed copse of trees. Most facilities like this one showed obvious signs of neglect: chipped concrete walls, crumbling stairwells, the occasional exposed pipe or wire. It was very unusual for clinics to possess even a single computer, let alone an Internet connection. Yet resident nurses and physicians often did their best to add a human touch, stationing a plant by the window or hanging a church calendar on the wall. A tall fence made of corrugated metal sheeting surrounded the small yard of the Kyiv clinic, providing room for a few sawhorse benches under the shade of a tree whose branches reached ambitiously over the fence toward the exterior yard. Inside, the long narrow building was divided straight down the middle by a single hallway. Doors led into the physicians' shared offices on the left and into the rooms where methadone was stored and distributed on the right. If there was any sort of lavatory or source of running water on the premises, I never saw them.

Some clinics did possess such facilities, but might have been better off without them. One of the most memorable examples I saw was an MAT clinic outside of Sevastopol, Crimea. It took me nearly two hours on two different bus lines to get there from the city center. I wondered whether the people receiving treatment spent their entire day going back and forth on that lengthy commute (some of my interviews would indicate that they did). The building itself was, in a word, brutalist: a thick-walled, three-story, concrete fortress that appeared partially abandoned and was clearly in disrepair. The walls hadn't seen a new coat of paint in at least ten years, and the yard appeared to have been left unswept and untended for even longer. Unlike the narcology clinic in Kyiv, this facility did have restrooms. I walked under leaky pipes through large patches of darkness in the basement to reach them. Many public restrooms in Ukraine still charge a nominal fee for entry and place a staff member near the door to distribute meager rations of toilet paper to patrons from the only available roll. As a frequent traveler, I had long made a habit of carrying tissues in my purse wherever I went, so I was not caught off guard when I reached the restroom in the clinic to find no toilet paper in sight. What did surprise me, though, were the supplies that had been left there in its place. A small wooden filing box had been drilled into the concrete wall where a toilet paper dispenser might have been. It was filled with square newspaper clippings. The newsprint was cheap. Ink rubbed off onto my fingertips as I leafed through the sheets to find that they were all daily crosswords puzzles. The nurses, it seemed, had deposited them there for reuse after they had exceeded their utility as pastimes.

Not all clinics were this bleak, however. The main MAT clinic in Odessa (one that opened *after* the cessation of the pilot project in the basement apartment downtown) occupied the opposite end of the spectrum. It was housed in a large TB hospital within walking distance of the central train station. The large verdant campus sat away from the street, backed up against one of the city's most idyllic beaches. On the grounds, a dozen or so stand-alone buildings surrounded a large, tree-filled courtyard—so large, in fact, that one could easily stroll along its manicured paths oblivious to the fact that an inpatient respiratory ward awaited just out of sight at the other end. The MAT clinic was located in a modest structure at the rear of the grounds. The clinic's head physician, a middle-aged woman named Alexandra Nikolaeva, saw patients in a series of small rooms outfitted with soft furniture and plenty of electric kettles for hot tea. She retained one of these rooms for her "private" office, though it hardly deserved the name. All day long, clients and

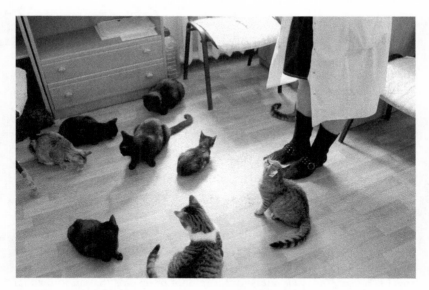

**Resident cats gather at Alexandra Nikolaeva's feet as she feeds them treats.
Photo by author.**

clinic nurses would pour in and out through her office door, which was always open. So, for that matter, were her office windows, with the result that stray cats residing on the hospital grounds took up sabbaticals of varied length near her radiator. When I first visited her office, I was startled to find no fewer than ten of them curled up on various chairs and bookshelves, which, by the looks of things, had long been surrendered for these purposes.

Alexandra was a highly competent physician and a loving individual. She took great care in creating a space where her patients could meet not only their health-care needs but also their emotional needs. She made sure that her patients knew each other's names. She organized birthday celebrations for family members and memorials for those who passed away. She encouraged patients to loiter around the clinic as often as they could to eat cookies, drink tea, and build deeper connections with the staff. She had earned a deep respect from the people she served. I interviewed more than half of her patients over the course of several long visits, and each one of them credited Alexandra with their ongoing health and well-being.

"This Is Not American Heroin"

The convivial atmosphere at the Odessa clinic fostered some of the most candid and fascinating conversations I had during my research in Ukraine. For example, it was in Alexandra's office, flanked by teakettles and snoozing cats, where I received my most thorough tutoring on the proper use of drug-related slang. *Shirka*, I learned, is the common name for the opiate solution most popular in Ukraine. A *chek* (adapted from *cheka*, another name for *shirka*) is a small bag or package of opiate product, the unit in which *shirka* and other street drugs were sold. The word *kaif* can be roughly translated as "a high." In the words of a young mother from this clinic, "we *narkomany* are always seeking some kind of *kaif*." Then there was the term *dozniak*, a word for which I have found no exact equivalent in English, though the concept certainly exists. From the root word *doza*, which in Russian and Ukrainian means "a dose," *dozniak* refers to the amount of opioids that an individual needs to consume in order to achieve *kaif*. In the general vernacular, the word *kaif* was used in manners that I found almost poetic. The term was often engaged in broader contexts to refer to satisfaction with one's life or even a physical sense of catharsis or release. "It's like when you get in a hot bath after working hard and getting really dirty," one of my research assistants explained, "Or when you've been on your feet all day in really high heels, and you come home and kick them off and rub your toes into the carpet." She rolled her eyes back in luxurious bliss. "Oh! Yes. That's *kaif*!"

This Odessan clinic is also where I received my first lessons in how locals produce the types of organic opiates that are sold by the *chek* around town. Sasha, a bright-eyed man in his forties who boasted several decades of experience injecting opioids was my most attentive tutor. "This is not American heroin," he said. "We have *shirka*. These are Ukrainian opiates. I produce it myself. I make it from poppies. I add two different components, an anhydride and a solvent, and I can make opiates for you that way. Me, myself. I would make opiates for you myself." He laughed. "In America, I know, you don't do this. But we are old, experienced *narkomany*. We do. Young folks don't know how to do it, but I'm a long-time user (Rus: *staryy narkoman*). I've been doing this since 1987."

The poppies that Sasha referred to have long been cultivated in Ukraine, Belarus, and parts of Russia. The seeds of this plant are a staple ingredient in Ukrainian cooking, used in an abundance of pastries and desserts. *Shirka*, by contrast, is typically produced by creating extracts from poppy-straw, the fibrous husk left behind after the flowering plant has been dried and the seeds removed from the pod. Some Ukrainians acquire *shirka* by harvesting their own poppy. This was evidenced by a particularly slow afternoon during the summer of 2013 spent at an outreach organization in Mykolaiv where I was supposed to be conducting interviews. "Sorry, there's no one here," the director told me apologetically, while serving me a third, conciliatory cup of tea. "Everyone must be out at the dacha [a country house] harvesting poppy!" Others purchase *shirka* on the street from those blessed with the energy or the resources to be so industrious. In 2013, the price of a single unit of this organic poppy straw derivative sold on the street ranged from UAH 60 (about USD 7.50 at the time of data collection) in Mykolaiv to upward of UAH 100 (about USD 12.50 at the time of data collection) in Sevastopol and L'viv.

Though the extraction of opiate solutions from poppy straw seems to fit neatly within more broadly held Ukrainian sensibilities about the superiority of organic or "natural" products, I frequently heard MAT patients voice a preference for the "clean" (Rus: *chistii*), synthetic narcotics available in hospital pharmacies, which they would contrast to the "dirty" (Rus: *griaznii*), organically-derived drugs available on the street. Sasha viewed this "cleanliness" as a benefit of the methadone he was receiving through Alexandra Nikolaeva. "[Methadone] is a switch to something better than those narcotics flowing around the streets here, which are more, like, they're dirty. From a medical perspective they're dirty drugs. So you come here [seeking treatment] because you're hung up [dependent] on this dirty swamp water." He, and many others, connected these difficulties to the poor quality of the drugs they had consumed. Sasha used such language ("dirty," "swampy," "mud") numerous times during our interviews to describe the substances he had consumed, in one form or another, almost daily since 1987. In the subsequent years, he had acquired (but also treated and successfully controlled) an HIV infection. He also had some scarring on his liver from heavy drinking—though this would hardly put him in the minority among Eastern European men his age. Overall, though, and despite his nearly three decades of opioid use, Sasha did not appear—to my eyes—to be that much worse for wear. His eyes were bright, his skin clear, his energy level high, his personality kind and bubbly. He did not display any of the outward signs of a sickly or "addicted" individual, which so many stereotypes and media images have taught us to expect, and I sometimes pondered how real his physical challenges really were.

On the other hand, though, Sasha had been injecting opioids since I was a child. His experience with opioids nearly outstrips my own experience of being alive. What capacity did I have to speak back to or contradict the knowledge he has gained from thousands of bodily encounters with opioids: the highs, the hangovers, the ease or the struggle of pushing the drug through a needle, the sting of the needle hitting his flesh, the calm in his muscles as the opioid attached to the receptors in his brain and set the activity in his central nervous system back a notch or two. Sasha was nothing if not a sophisticate about the neurochemical romance forged between different opioids and his own body, and he used this deeply personal knowledge to manage his body with methadone and chemically protect his sense of self the best way he knew how.

To those readers without a personal history of substance use or chemical dependency, this claim that Sasha stuck to his methadone treatment in order to protect his sense of self may sound odd. But consider this: social and biomedical research has produced a mountain of evidence indicating that habitual use of illicit opioids, like that in which Sasha had engaged, is most often shaped by the need to stave off withdrawal symptoms and feel "normal," not by uncontrolled impulses or an overpowering desire to get "high." In fact, researchers have been making this observation since the 1940s. In his groundbreaking 1947 book *Opiate Addiction*, Chicago sociologist Alfred Lindesmith argued, "Persons become addicts when they recognize or perceive the significance of the withdrawal distress that they are experiencing, and if they do not recognize withdrawal distress, they do not become addicts, regardless of other circumstances" (1947, 8). A few years later, Howard Becker's (1953) ethnography on marijuana smoking highlighted a similar facet of substance use: not only withdrawal symptoms, as Lindesmith argued, but also the sensations of euphoria that a drug may bring are learned interpretations of the drug's neurochemical effects. If this is true of illicit drugs, then it can be true of any substance, and if it can be true of any substance, this opens our lived experiences to all variety of subtle chemical manipulations of our alertness, anxiety, and other physical and psychological states.

This chemical malleability of our physical and psychological states is precisely what sociologist Nikolas Rose meant when he wrote about the use of "smart" antidepressant drugs, like Prozac, for the creation of "neurochemical selves": "[Such] drugs promise to help the individual him or herself, in alliance with the doctor and the molecule, to discover the intervention that will address precisely a specific molecular anomaly at the root of something that personally troubles the individual concerned and disrupts his or her life, in order to restore the self to its life, and itself, again" (Rose 2007, 203). Or, to quote Michel Foucault, who put it much more succinctly, this is "the way a human being turns himself [or herself] into a subject" (1982, 778). In this view, where we may think of all humans as engaged in the chemical manipulation of their bodies through food, drink, medications, and other activities, we could say that Sasha returns to himself by taking his methadone in the same way that I return to my own self by drinking two (or more) cups of coffee every morning. I do not think these ritual, chemical manipulations are truly all that different at their base.

Local Epidemics

Like all human behaviors, substance use practices—whether they involve smoking marijuana, drinking whiskey, or injecting opioids—and the risks that accompany them are shaped by the social environments in which they take place. Medical anthropologist Philippe Bourgois, who has conducted some of the most prominent work on the social aspects of substance use in the United States, has even considered the implications of perceiving people who use drugs as their own social class. In his photo ethnography of homeless adults living near San Francisco (a collaboration with photographer Jeffrey Schonberg), Bourgois offered a deeply intimate picture of the "moral economy of sharing" that shaped heroin use in this community (Bourgois and Schonberg 2009). He argued, for example, that the combination of local ethics and interpersonal relationships oblige those engaging in heroin use to share injection equipment (like cookers and cottons) and assist each other when one of them was feeling "dopesick." Even the common practice of cooperating to buy and share bags of heroin, he argued, formed "the basis for sociality and establishes boundaries of [social] networks that provide companionship and also facilitate material survival" (2009, 83). The patterns of heroin use in this community did not—and could not—make sense outside of the social context in which that use took place. The way opioids interacted with the neuroreceptors in these individuals' brains was arguably a purely biochemical phenomenon, but all other aspects of their heroin use were anything but.

In my own research into illicit opioid use in Rhode Island, which I conducted as I was writing this book, I found that many people who use opioids relied on trusted social relationships to organize their own experiences of substance use and to navigate the risks posed by strong, synthetic opioids like fentanyl in the local drug market (Carroll et al. 2017). The moral economy of heroin use in Rhode Island obliged practices such as people in treatment sharing their prescribed buprenorphine with someone who was still using but experiencing severe withdrawal (even if that person was a stranger); friends and significant others acting as accountability partners to remember to take test hits and control their level of heroin use; and low-level drug suppliers informing their clients if fentanyl was found to be in their product. I was even aware of an occasion when a low-level dealer called one of his clients to ask her to bring the overdose-reversing drug naloxone to assist a different client whom he was with who was, at that moment, overdosing. Here, the local culture and the intimate social networks that grew from it held considerable influence over not simply what types of drugs people used or how they used them, but over the local risk environment. This led patterns of opioid overdose to conform closely to the shape of these social networks and the relationships of mutual assistance that residents had forged.

Similarly, most of the MAT patients I met in Ukraine not only made a practice of using opiates in trusted settings, but were also initiated into substance use through intimate social networks. Mariya, a woman in her early thirties receiving methadone at the narcology clinic in Kyiv, began using *shirka* with a boyfriend to blow off steam. "It just makes everything soft around the edges," she told me. "It's all just to relax right?" I met another young man in his early twenties at a community center in Sevastopol who recounted the story of his friends putting codeine solution into a soda for him to drink. Though he never admitted to feeling pressured, something in the way he told this story made me suspect that a certain element of "come on, everyone else is doing it" lay underneath his decision to take those first gulps.

Many Ukrainians' initiation into alcohol or substance use is a similar social process. This is true, first and foremost, because so much of public life in Ukraine is already deeply invested in peer groups and the social consumption of other drugs, especially alcohol, within those groups. From early childhood, for example, Ukrainian schoolchildren generally attend classes in a single classroom year after year, staying with the same students until graduation. Anthropologist Anna Fournier has observed that these school-based peer groups (sometimes referred to by the Russian term *odnoklassniki*, which can be roughly translated as "classmates") were once governed through "horizontal surveillance": a culture of self-policing among peers that was actively promoted among Soviet youth in order to engender the proper orientation toward the social collective (Fournier 2012). Fournier argues that since Ukraine's independence this form of social policing has given way to principles of self-knowledge and self-development, encouraging the development of a more individualized (or "decollectivized") personhood in the classroom; however, descriptions of adolescent social life offered to me by my own friends in Ukraine indicate that pressures to conform to the collective will of one's peer group remain remarkably strong even today. For many, these were the only social networks they had access to during their youth. Falling out of favor with that group would mean spending the remainder of your adolescence as a social outcast. Thus, one could say that peer pressure likely played a role in many Ukrainians' initiation into substance use; at the same time, it may be equally appropriate to question whether deviating from the norms of the group was even conceivable in the first place.

Though biomedical treatments for opioid use disorder, like MAT, are designed to intervene on individuals in isolation from their surrounding environment, the social aspect would frequently rear its head in even the most personal clinical moments. One particular occasion, which stands out in my memory, took place in the summer of 2014. I was shadowing outreach workers from L'viv as they journeyed into the villages surrounding the city to provide syringe access, counseling, and a variety of other services to people who used drugs in the rural parts of the region. On that day, a nurse had joined the outreach team and was offering rapid tests for various infections to any participants who were interested. The test, itself, was a clever device. It consisted of a plastic dish with five small wells, which allowed drops of blood to be placed and wicked up into strips of litmus-like paper that revealed test results in a series of windows cut into the plastic for viewing. The test screened for four communicable infections at once: HIV, hepatitis A, hepatitis C, and syphilis. To preserve patient confidentiality, the nurse conducted these screenings and gave test results in a small compartment at the back of the bus we had driven into the village.

Toward the end of the day, the nurse agreed to show me one of the many tests she had completed, never revealing to me whose test I was viewing. The

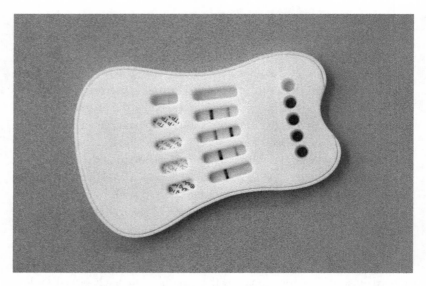

A rapid test, used by the outreach organization in L'viv, which screens for hepatitis A, hepatitis C, HIV, and syphilis. Photo by author.

little windows revealed positive results for HIV, hepatitis A, and hepatitis C. The syphilis test was negative. The nurse pointed to the syphilis result saying, "We didn't have many today. We rarely do. When we have positives for syphilis, almost everyone that day is positive." She went on to explain that viral infections like HIV and hepatitis were so common among program participants that a slate-full of negative results would be something of an anomaly. Syphilis, however, tended to appear largely within tight-knit social groups, as it is transmitted sexually rather than through the sharing of injection equipment. Networks of intimate social relationships often include some arrangement of sexual relationships as well. A positive syphilis test, therefore, likely indicates less about an individual's substance use or other risky behaviors than about the size and the composition of the peer groups into which those behaviors are embedded.

In addition to the social drivers of substance use and related risks, many individuals who use drugs in Ukraine face an array of biological risks for illness and infection that were beyond the influence of the social and beyond their individual ability to control. Arguably the most perilous of these is TB, a bacterial infection that can be extremely difficult to treat and is endemic in Ukraine. Recent estimates suggest that approximately 90 out of every 100,000 people in Ukraine (or approximately 40,000 people) become newly infected with TB each year (WHO Regional Office for Europe 2017). In the human body, TB mycobacterium has a synergistic relationship with HIV. This means that each of these diseases makes its host more susceptible to infection by the other. They also speed up each other's progression toward advanced disease when someone is coinfected (WHO 2004b). Poverty, incarceration, and frail health-care systems have also long conspired to cause higher rates of TB among drug-using populations in Eastern Europe (Acosta et al. 2014; Orcau, Caylà, and Martínez 2011; Stuckler et al. 2008). Consequently, public health research carried out in 2005 indicated that the risk of TB infection was more than thirty times higher among Ukrainians who inject drugs than among their noninjecting counterparts at that time (van der Werf et al. 2006), mirroring the high rates of HIV among people who inject drugs in Ukraine.

In addition to the social aspects of substance use and the biological mechanisms by which certain infectious diseases interact, there is a third factor that shapes these behaviors and the risks that accompany them: the material technology of substance use. By "material technology" I mean, in part, the very drugs that are being used. The importance of this material technology to the shape of local epidemics is well-demonstrated by a large ethnographic and epidemiological study conducted in Philadelphia in 2012. This study found that two different kinds of heroin—Colombian white powder and Mexican black tar—were circulating in the city, but that access to these two varieties was not equally distributed among all residents; Hispanic and white residents predominantly bought heroin from Hispanic and white dealers, who sold heroin of Colombian origin, whereas African American residents primarily bought heroin from African American dealers, who largely sold heroin of Mexican origin (Rosenblum et al. 2014). These two separate but overlapping heroin markets presented different types of risk and altered the consequences of heroin use for each set of consumers. White powder heroin is easy to dissolve and cook, but also very easy to "cut" with other products (with other opioids like fentanyl or with "filler" products like talcum powder or mannitol). Black tar, on the other hand, is harder to cut and therefore generally less adulterated by mid-level suppliers, but it is also harder to prepare for injection and manipulate with a syringe. As a result, the use of black tar heroin is associated with higher rates of infection, abscess, and soft tissue injury, but lower rates of HIV and accidental overdose (Ciccarone 2009; Mars et al. 2015).

In Ukraine, very little heroin is made available to the people I worked with at MAT clinics. As described above, most people make their own *shirka* or produce various opioid solutions from pharmaceutical products at home. In some cases, people will seek opioid products from pharmacies, including cough syrups, cold medicines, and pain medications with codeine, just to name a few. Often the intention is simply to ingest these medications orally to self-medicate withdrawal symptoms associated with opioid use disorder. For this reason, it is challenging to isolate particular risks or injuries that stem from the use of opioids from different sources in Ukraine. One noteworthy exception, however, involves the process of removing the inert ingredients from these pharmaceutical products, isolating the codeine, and synthesizing it into desomorphine. The resulting, injectable liquid desomorphine solution is known as *krokodil* or, simply, *krok*. *Krok* has received a significant amount of media attention in recent years, due largely to its association with rapid and extensive tissue damage (Laessig 2011; Shuster 2013; Walker 2011; "'Zombie Apocalypse' in Russia" 2012). Synthesizing *krok* is not easy in the best of circumstances, and serious nerve and tissue damage can occur if the solutions injected are too acidic or contain other harmful, residual substances (Grund, Latypov, and Harris 2013). These injuries have given *krok* its nefarious reputation in popular media. However, based on the apparent prevalence of this practice, as indicated by my interviews with many individuals who have used *krok*, it is clear that not all who use desomorphine experience these negative physical effects.

The "material technologies" of substance use also include the tools used to prepare and consume them (i.e., smoke, snort, inject). In Ukraine, it is the types of needles and syringes available that are arguably of the most consequence. In the United States, people who consume opioids and other substances intravenously (as opposed to alternative injection practices like "muscling" or "skin popping," both of which involve injecting into soft tissue rather than into a vein) often use 28- or 29-gauge tuberculin syringes. These are the same as those commonly used by diabetics to inject insulin: small, disposable syringes equipped with a narrow needle (good for targeting delicate blood vessels) and a barrel that holds 1 milliliter (mL) of fluid. These syringes are stocked in almost every syringe access program in the United States and are preferred by the majority of clients at every U.S. syringe access program in which I have ever worked. In contrast, injecting *shirka* requires a syringe with a very large barrel. In its prepared form, *shirka* is a dilute opiate solution. One needs to inject a greater volume of this product than is required of more potent opioid solutions like heroin—often upward of 5 mL or even 10 mL of fluid.

This difference in syringe volume has major implications for the risk of disease transmission. Small amounts of blood are commonly drawn up into a syringe before injection. In U.S. medical settings, this is sometimes called "flash" and is used to ensure that the needle is seated properly in a vein. More volume inside the barrel of the syringe means more space for blood to enter, mix with the substance being injected, and contaminate the inside of the barrel. Large barrel syringes also typically have a large "dead space," the cavity found in the interior of the needle and the well at the bottom of the barrel that retains small amounts of fluid even when the plunger is fully depressed. More dead space means more residual, potentially contaminated fluid after an injection, and more residual, contaminated fluid means higher chances of disease transmission if that syringe is shared or reused (Zule 2012). The risks posed by dead space have been greatly reduced in many smaller varieties of syringe, for which low dead space models have been developed (Vickerman, Martin, and Hickman 2013). Large volume syringes have undergone no such technological overhaul, despite the fact that syringe sharing has long been common practice in Ukraine (Booth et al. 2003).

Though these descriptions paint a dire portrait of the risks faced by Ukrainians who use drugs, it is important to keep in mind that people never set out with the intention of developing a substance use disorder or of acquiring HIV or hepatitis infections. Mariya, from the clinic in Kyiv, was still conducting a personal accounting of her history and developing an understanding of how her life went in the direction it did, even years into her successful treatment with methadone. "When I started [using drugs]," she told me, "we had no *narkomany* in our village. I had no idea that I would end up like this, living the life that I'm living now." I have heard many individuals—American and Ukrainian—laugh off such comments. To those who find the risks posed by substance use so untenable that they would never dream of using, the suggestion that someone who did use might not have seen bad outcomes approaching may appear genuinely absurd. The story that Mariya told, however, reminded me of so many of my own failures. Once I had arrived at them, I hardly knew how I had arrived there, recognizing only that something big about my situation needed to change. Similarly, many Ukrainians who seek treatment at MAT clinics do so not simply to return themselves to physical health but also to rid themselves of the destructive social and material milieus that have shaped their substance use. Many hope MAT will provide that "something big" to help get them back to where they want to be.

Medication-Assisted Treatment

As I was conducting the bulk of my research in Ukraine, approximately 8,000 people were receiving MAT for opioid use disorder—less than 3 percent of the estimated 310,000 Ukrainians who inject drugs (Bojko et al. 2015). Since space in treatment programs was at such a premium, I wanted to understand what was leading certain people to opt in to MAT and others to opt out. This was, in fact, the original motivating question of my research: why did people who use opioids in Ukraine decide to begin MAT in the first place? The question was premised on the understanding that enrolling in MAT presented significant challenges. In addition to chemically "chaining" patients to their clinic, where they had to appear every single day to receive their medication, enrollment in MAT also required that patients be listed on a national registry of known "addicts." Appearing on the registry stripped them of the right to obtain a gun permit or a driver's license, hold certain occupations, and travel abroad—though the latter would hardly have been feasible anyway, given their medication needs. In light of the significant sacrifices that must be made, did enrolling in MAT really appear better than the alternative?

I very quickly learned that MAT patients in Ukraine asked themselves many of the same questions. This first became apparent on a hot, sunny day at the narcology clinic in Kyiv. Not long after I arrived for observations that day, a young man in a panama hat and a five-day shadow took notice of me. As I settled into a space in the shade where several men seemed mesmerized by an ongoing backgammon game, he turned, tilted his head to look over the smoke streaming from the cigarette in his mouth, and asked, "Who are you?" He squinted at me with suspicion, clearly sussing me out as the interloper I was. I introduced myself as an American researcher. I explained that I had spent a long time working in various programs for people who use drugs in the United States and was now interested in how such programs operated in Ukraine. He sat up, eyes wide. "Oh. Fascinating," he mumbled. He pursed his lips around his cigarette and shuffled over from his bench to the spot right next to me. He introduced himself as Maksim and began asking me questions.

"Do doctors in the U.S. give out methadone in tablets or in liquid form?"

"Can a person get methadone by prescription and pick it up at the pharmacy?"

"Are there supervised injection sites in the U.S.?"

"How much money do your doctors make?"

"Do you have incentive programs that pay people to take methadone?"

"Are people who use drugs allowed to get driver's licenses?"

"Can the police just throw you in jail and forget about you?"

"How do doctors treat people who use drugs?"

"And pregnant women who use? What happens to them?"

I answered each one as best I could, and found myself ruminating long after on what this series of questions revealed about Maksim's life. A close read of many of his prompts reveals a very personal reckoning with the social milieu of substance use in Ukraine. Other questions in his litany revealed an ambivalence about the treatment he was receiving. As we talked, I learned that Maksim had been taking methadone for nearly eight years. That made him one of the most experienced patients in the program.

"Do you still like it, after all this time?" I asked.

"Well," he said, "I long ago realized that I'm an 'addict.' That's just how it is (Rus: *Ya—narkoman. Vot eto vot*). If I didn't come here, where would I be? Back in prison or something. I've already been there three times." He held up three fingers in front of his face.

MAT patients, including Maksim, overwhelmingly reported that they stay in treatment in their respective MAT programs because they value the long-term physical stability it provides. That stability does not come simply from the consistent availability of methadone, reducing the daily hustle to find opioids and stave off withdrawal; the methadone also helps stabilize him physically, leaving his brain and his body feeling calmer than when he was using *shirka* every day. Vincent Dole, Marie Nyswander, and Mary Jeanne Kreek, three physicians who ran the first clinical trial for MAT with methadone in the United States, coined the term "narcotic blockade" to describe this stabilization effect (1966). In one of their seminal articles based on this research, they outlined three different "states" that an individual with opioid dependency might be experiencing at any given time: "high," when someone has consumed enough opioids to feel sedated and even possibly euphoric; "sick," or "abstinence," when someone is experiencing physical withdrawal symptoms; and "straight," a neutral territory that falls somewhere in between the other two (1966). "Straight" is when people have a level of opioids in their blood stream that is neither too high nor too low, when they are experiencing neither the physical effects of withdrawal nor the psychological effects of a high. Feeling "straight" is the same thing as feeling "normal." People who develop opioid dependence and use opioids regularly often find themselves swinging back and forth between "sick" and "high."

Medications used in MAT stabilize patients in a "normal" mode of functioning by "blocking" the brain's ability to feel high or fall into withdrawal. This "narcotic blockade" effect is made possible by chemical differences between many illicit opioids and MAT medications. Opioid agonist medications for MAT, like methadone and buprenorphine, bind with receptors in the brain just as other narcotics like heroin, morphine, and *shirka* do, but, unlike these other drugs, methadone and buprenorphine stay in the body much longer. In general, the effects of heroin and many other organic opiates in the body begin to wear off after about four or five hours (Field et al. 2012). Methadone, by contrast, confers effects that can last up to twenty-four hours in an opioid-tolerant patient (Grissinger 2011), and the effects of buprenorphine, when administered correctly, can last even longer (Welsh and Valadez-Meltzer 2005). These lasting effects prevent MAT patients from falling back into withdrawal every few hours, as they often do when using heroin or *shirka*. Furthermore, the relative "strength" with which both of these medications attach to the opioid receptors in the brain (called "binding affinity") is high, which prevents most MAT patients from experiencing a sense of euphoria if they use illicit drugs while on their medication. The illicit drugs will not be strong enough to take the place of MAT medications on these receptors. Thus, as Maksim and so many other individuals who participated in my research attested, MAT is not simply a substitute narcotic that replaces one "addiction" for another. Regular *shirka* use is defined by a constant struggle to maintain a sense of self and a sense of control. MAT, on the other hand, is not. Risks are low. Stability is high. Success rates are impressive compared with other forms of treatment. These features have helped lift MAT to the status of a "gold standard" for treating opioid use disorder in the eyes of the international medical community.

Maksim's very positive experience with MAT is, of course, not universal. Not all bodies are the same; nor are all experiences with opioid-agonist MAT comparable. Some people do not tolerate methadone well. Some feel ill or groggy while taking it. I have known people who experienced severe nausea while taking buprenorphine. Perhaps some readers of this book have taken MAT to treat opioid use disorder and find my description of Maksim's treatment experiences, above, to be inconsistent with their own. These variations are real, and no treatment is ideal for every body. Nevertheless, clinical research has consistently found MAT to be the most universally effective way to treat opioid use disorder, prevent opioid overdose, and reduce the use of illegal narcotics among those who are attempting to quit (Mattick et al. 2009, 2014).

Patients like Maksim may receive either methadone or buprenorphine as part of their treatment regimen. Both are approved for use in MAT in Ukraine. Methadone is sold commercially under several brand names. At the time of my research, two varieties were available: Methaddict®, produced by the German company Sandoz Pharmaceuticals GmbH, and Metadol®, produced by Paladin Labs in Canada. Buprenorphine was available under the brand name Addnok®, produced by Basic Pharma manufacturing B. V. in the Netherlands. (In the United States, buprenorphine formulations are frequently sold under the brand names Subutex® or Suboxone®. These brand names may be more familiar to some readers.) Each MAT clinic in Ukraine is typically stocked with only one of these medications, not both. This is because the daily operation of MAT clinics is overseen not by the MoH itself but by regional health councils that operate relatively independently under the aegis of the MoH. In practice, this means that regional councils have the legal authority to stock clinics within their region with both methadone and buprenorphine; however, they are not required to stock both simultaneously, and obtaining both medications requires more paperwork, more time, and more money. As a result, few MAT patients have personal experience with more than one of these drugs. This allows MAT patients and their social networks to develop a collectively deep but individually narrow understanding of MAT drugs and their effects.

Patients' efforts to construct or improve their social selves were readily apparent in the treatment goals they had set for themselves when entering MAT programs. These treatment plans varied. Some patients managed to lower their dose of MAT drugs and eventually quit the program. This outcome would have represented the ultimate bodily freedom—from opioids and from the clinic. It is a tough goal to achieve, though. Opioid use disorder is driven by more than simple chemical dependency, and using MAT medications as a short-term step-down tool does not resolve any of those underlying causes. Most clinicians I spoke to were able to report that between two and four patients had "left" their program in the previous year (though some of them, it seemed, always came back). Other patients said that they wanted to quit methadone eventually but did not feel ready. Many expressed a significant amount of anxiety over quitting MAT. Some feared the difficult withdrawal from methadone, which is largely understood to be stronger than withdrawal from *shirka*. A man on MAT in Sevastopol voiced this concern, "People are going from these easy drugs like *shirka* and heroin to methadone. It's harder to quit, you know? I know people who have quit methadone, but it cost them a lot of energy, a lot of health. You have to understand that people here are not healthy, and when they withdraw, their diseases can appear, can flare up really badly, so quitting can be dangerous." Others feared that they would return to street drugs and, as a result end up sick, in jail, or dead. For them, returning to methadone seemed a more reasonable coping mechanism following a relapse than returning to street drugs, which makes quitting methadone in the first place seem rather illogical to them. "In any case, sooner or later, we all come back," explained Vova, a young man receiving MAT in Simferopol, Crimea. "There is some kind of thing that is stuck [in us] that becomes hard to cope with (Rus: *Gde-to tam sidit kakoi-to klin s kotorym spravitsia ne tak legko*)."

Many MAT patients found this a reasonable trade-off for the benefits that treatment offered them. In the words of a middle-aged man who received methadone from a clinic in L'viv, "The benefits of the program are this: I'm not running around. I'm not in jail. I don't have problems with the police. I'm feeling calm in the mornings. My mornings have become so peaceful." Others specifically praised the efficiency of the program. Many MAT patients delighted in telling me how quickly they were in and out of the clinic each day. "It's great," a young woman in Odessa told me, echoing the answers of many other patients I had talked to. "I come here, say hello, take my pills, head out the door, and I'm home and ready to start my day by 9:30 A.M." A young man from L'viv excitedly told me, "I've been here for four years and

I've never had problems with the law! I don't use illegal drugs, the dose that I get here is enough for me. The tablets hold me up. I feel totally normal."

Not all views were this rosy, however. Oksana, a woman in her late twenties who received methadone at the brutalist, concrete MAT clinic in Sevastopol, was one of several patients I met who were dissatisfied with what their efforts to initiate MAT had gained them:

JC: So how long have you been coming here to this [methadone] program?

O: Two and a half years.

JC: And where did you first hear about the program?

O: From a girlfriend.

JC: She was a patient here?

O: Yea.

JC: And what did she tell you about being treated here?

O: That she had so much free time, you know. She's got work and her kids, and she can take care of those things properly. She said she liked the program.

JC: And do you like the program?

O: See, for me, it's like this. I came here for the first time, and they were like, "Oh, we'll help you." But people are just coming here and they keep coming. The problem here is that there is no detox facility. There is no way to quit the program. I decided that I wanted to quit—to quit the methadone. I talked to the narcologist about this, asking them to lower my dose so that I could quit, and they said, "Why? Why is this something you want to do on your own?" And they wouldn't decrease my dose. So, in reality, there is no possibility of quitting. And, you know, earlier, I was on Metadol®. I took 25–30 mg of that. Here, they started me on Methaddict®. I'm taking 80 mg of that. I don't feel good on Methaddict®. They have to give you a dose that's twice as high.

JC: So, if you could go back to before you started the program, if you had the choice to make all over again, whether to start this program, would you make the same decision?

O: No. No . . .

Oksana's frustration left a strong impression. My memory of this conversation served as a constant reminder that every treatment slot and outcome statistic represented a unique human being. All of these people possessed unique bodies, preferences, concerns, and goals. Yet, even in her discontent, Oksana's story also testifies to the most common trait that so many MAT patients had in common. Namely, the reasons voiced by most for seeking out MAT were similar to their reasons for initiating substance use in the first place: they were social in nature. Maksim told me his parents had convinced him to start treatment. Others were encouraged by friends or significant others. Some were convinced to begin MAT by peers who were already receiving this form of care. Those who decided to seek MAT were very likely already contemplating making some sort of move toward change. The centrality of social ties to so many treatment-seeking narratives reveals how closely this decision is often linked to what Nikolas Rose called "restoring the self to life, and itself, again" (2007).

Where We Go from Here

Through an ethnographic accounting of opioid use in Ukraine, this chapter has detailed, first, how this region of the globe, with its unique political and cultural history, has produced its own "homegrown" culture of substance use and spectrum of substance use practices. Second, the chapter has described the local characteristics that render Ukraine an ideal setting for asking the questions posed in the Introduction of this book. In particular, the unusual economic, political, and epidemiological features of contemporary Ukraine put many of the fundamental assumptions that guide the logic of contemporary global health under duress. The internationally dominant biomedical approach, which serves as the foundational logic of MAT as promoted by groups like the Global Fund, has effectively reinforced the moral principles that have framed addiction for much of the twentieth century: namely, that compulsive substance use is caused by a deficiency of the will (Valverde 1998). As a result, the social imagination of drug use and "addiction" in many parts of the world typically places blame for the myriad harms resulting from drug use onto the very individuals who use, selectively pathologizing people who use drugs according to the models by which choice, control, desire, bodily health, and psychological well-being are understood in each place. The post-Soviet sphere, with its long legacy of socially oriented medicine and narcological approaches to substance use, places a particularly illuminating pressure on the philosophies embodied by international global health projects.

The following chapters of this book explore what may occur and what is at stake when new biomedical technologies, such as MAT, are deployed in diverse regions of the world without a firm understanding of how those technologies will interact with local systems of meaning. I follow previous insights from scholars of the post-Soviet sphere who have highlighted the poor fit between the economic priorities demanded by international development projects and the financial realities being faced by client nations (Hrycak 2007; Keshavjee 2014; Koch 2013; Phillips 2008), as well as those who point to the broader political consequences of putting destabilized nations in the position of receiving aid in the first place (Driscoll 2015). Ironically, both of these phenomena can negatively affect the democratic projects that international donors otherwise seek to promote. With Ukraine now fully entangled in the global economy and often caught in the middle of political jockeying between Europe and Russia, differences in such things as financial reasoning, understandings of state sovereignty, and social attitudes toward substance use behaviors can all illuminate features of the social and political substrate of the contemporary world. This matters not only for global health practice but also for our understanding of nation-building strategies in this region. These differences bring to light, especially, the ways in which the marginalization of people who use drugs has become a vital element in the social fabric of the former Soviet sphere.

Chapter 2

What Counts When You're Counting

In April 2007, in a leafy park dedicated to the Soviet cosmonauts, I met Gennadiy. He was a sharply dressed, university-educated man in his mid-twenties and the manager of a Global Fund–supported harm reduction program called "Better Together" in Odessa, Ukraine. A month earlier, I had written to him, introducing myself as an American social scientist who wanted to know more about Global Fund–supported harm reduction programs and how they were implemented in Ukraine. Gennadiy invited me to come visit and observe his operations for as long as I wished. He was visibly enthusiastic about his work and apparently undeterred by the potential bother of a curious foreigner poking around. A few weeks later, I traveled more than thirty hours by train from Budapest, Hungary, where I was living at the time, to accept his offer.

Long before I began this voyage—the first of many—into Ukraine, I worked for several years in a syringe access program in Portland, Oregon. I was, by that time, quite familiar with the politics of harm reduction in the United States. I was also accustomed to the consumer-services model of harm reduction that was, and still is, common in the United States, wherein people who inject drugs must present themselves at designated service points to receive the benefits of a program, acting as free-market consumers of their own health. I had also normalized to certain politically motivated regulations imposed on U.S. syringe access programs, such as the one-for-one rule, which stipulates that a used needle must be surrendered for a client to earn the right to receive a new one, as well as hard limits on the number of syringes that any one client could receive on a single visit. Even though researchers have found this kind of one-for-one exchange to be much less effective at preventing disease than no-strings-attached syringe access programs (Bluthenthal et al. 2007), such counterproductive rules often flourish amid empty promises from politicians or public health authorities to be tough on drug use or reduce needle litter on the street. Much of the harm reduction work done in Eastern Europe—especially in 2007, when I first visited Better Together—was cultivated by industry leaders, like staff at the Alliance, to mirror the standards and practices first developed and implemented in Western Europe (the Netherlands in particular) and the West Coast of North America (in major cities like Seattle, San Francisco, and Vancouver). Better Together, therefore, had much in common with the programs I knew from back home. At one point, the thought even occurred to me that were there not signs and posters in Russian on the wall, I might have reasonably concluded that I was still in Oregon.

Better Together offered a variety of services: from syringe access and legal advocacy to medical counseling and social support. The jewel in their crown was a buprenorphine-based MAT program, one of the first pilots in the country, which they helped operate out of a nondescript basement on the north end of town. I accompanied Better Together's outreach workers to this clinic often. Most were MAT patients, themselves, and would stop by to take their dose each day before their shifts began. Each time I went, I was surprised by how many bodies could be pressed into the clinic's cramped interior. In stark contrast to the open parks and breezy corridors of the nearby polyclinic and TB hospital—also frequent stops for the outreach staff—this place confronted visitors with tiny rooms, low ceilings, and narrow doors. The truth is, this was never meant to be a clinic. It was an ordinary commercial space like those often leased by small print shops and Internet cafés. It was a temporary home for a temporary program—a trial phase of what would grow into Ukraine's countrywide network of MAT clinics.

The syringe access program housed in Better Together's main office kept regular business hours. The staff followed a protocol I knew well: clients signed in when they arrived; one needle in for one needle out; no more than ten syringes per client per day. The syringe access program I worked for in Oregon also operated under one-for-one regulations. These rules were a constant source of difficulty for our clients, who were often unable to carry containers of dirty needles with them to our office. The mountains of paperwork maintained by the staff at Better Together's syringe access program also mirrored my experience in the United States. Every syringe had to be tracked: when it arrived, when it was distributed, to whom it went. The staff in Gennadiy's office kept these records diligently, putting pen to paper with each new visitor, perpetually fine-tuning totals on elaborate scrolls of spreadsheets crammed amid the clutter on their one, tiny desk.

This detailed record keeping served as an "obligatory passage point" (Callon 1986, 204) for the Global Fund and its contractors, a procedural element that allows these disparate entities to "talk" to each other through paperwork and data. Even though the staff of Better Together operated within a professional culture that reflected Ukrainian (and Odessan) values (Carroll 2011), and even as the staff members were largely free to pursue their own politics in advocating for local clients, there was nevertheless the need for clearly demarcated intersections where the activities of local actors like Better Together, national actors like the Alliance, and international actors like the Global Fund converge to generate a coherent and coordinated project. The data collected by Better Together's staff, destined for repackaging by the Alliance's accountants and delivery to the Global Fund for review, was one such point of convergence. Detailed monitoring has always been a keystone in the Global Fund's plan to reproduce internationally accepted standards of public health practice wherever their funds circulate. In a practical sense, this constant monitoring is useful for capturing key data about the efficacy of harm reduction efforts in Ukraine and the kinds of populations those efforts are able to reach. On a more abstract level, standardized reporting provides directors of Global Fund–supported programs with a common language through which the priorities of their funder can be communicated—as can individual organizations' conformity or resistance to that agenda. It thus reflects the audit culture that shapes business practices across much of Western Europe and North America.

These standardized reporting practices and the data such practices produce in Ukraine's internationally funded harm reduction world shape how people who use drugs, writ large, are conceived as specific "publics." In fact, different data collection regimes frame people who use drugs as a variety of different publics that appear to require different strategies for governing according to the values they are assigned within, or in relation to, political imaginations of the Ukrainian citizenry. Through its own monitoring and reporting practices, the Global Fund characterizes drug-using Ukrainians not as a true public (i.e., not as the "public" that is invoked by the term "public health"), but as a unique counterpublic: a delineated segment of social actors defined by common features, addressed through standardized discourse and practice, and "defined by [its] tension with a larger public," one of marked (and, in this case, inferior) social status (Warner 2002, 56). Whether or not Ukrainians who use drugs perceive themselves as a participatory public with a shared subculture that promotes alternative forms of citizenship, as Michael Warner originally defined the term (2002), the auditing practices of the Global Fund and its local subcontractors operate as though this is precisely what they are.

In considering the construction of this and other publics, I take as my premise the view long advanced by scholars of science and technology studies that all forms of knowledge production operate by bringing different actors into a set of social relations with one another. To create knowledge, in other words, one must create social ties—and occasionally break some as well. By virtue of their financial and legal entanglements with multiple authorities, local clinics and nongovernmental organizations (NGOs) often find themselves producing several, sometimes redundant, sometimes contradictory, sets of surveillance data about their clients—rendering them visible and governable by different authorities in different ways. In contrast to scholarship that casts international health projects as hegemonic forces with the capacity to overwhelm local power structures—as Johanna Tayloe Crane (2013) has argued Western academic institutions have done to health-care systems in Africa, for example, and as Salman Keshavjee (2014) has argued that neoliberal financial institutions have done to health-care systems in Central Asia—organizations like Better Together are able to thrive thanks to their ability to skillfully manage their entanglement in two distinct socioscientific networks: one dominated by the Global Fund, the other by the

Ukrainian Ministry of Health (MoH). Though both of these authoritative institutions are interested in monitoring the operation of harm reduction programs and services for people who use drugs, they nevertheless mandate different reporting practices in pursuit of very different goals. These divergent goals are, in turn, motivated by fundamentally different perceptions of who people who use drugs are and how medical and state institutions are obligated to respond to them.

Ultimately, through their entanglement in multiple, overlapping sociosci-entific networks guided by differing political goals, harm reduction programs for people who use drugs in Ukraine engage in multiple, simultaneous forms of governance over drug-using bodies. These coexisting modes of surveil-lance and control do not exist in conflict with each other so much as they succeed in integrating themselves into each other, becoming mutually sub-sumed through the course of daily clinical practice into a chimeric instrument of biopower that answers simultaneously to these two different sovereign au-thorities. In other words, a single monitoring paradigm can be manipulated to serve the goals of two different masters. Both of these surveillance projects are carried out, in part, through bureaucratic means, such as detailed clients logs and clinic records, but are oriented toward fundamentally incompatible institutional goals. Organizations like Better Together code-switch between these two discursive fields in order to remain in good standing with both au-thorities and, ultimately, to keep their doors open, participating in multiple modes of governmentality over people who use drugs as they do so.

Enrole Actors, Make Subjects

A common critique of global health interventions asserts that these projects serve to promote a specific set of neoliberal values—especially individual responsibility, personal ownership, and the utility of bureaucratization. Fueled by the idea that "participation in markets [is] an economic form of po-litical democracy" (Keshavjee 2014, 7), many global health interventions also seek to improve health outcomes by altering the relationships of health-care systems and individual citizens to the market economy through the imple-mentation of structural adjustment programs (SAPs) and fee-for-service med-ical care (Pfeiffer and Chapman 2010). These programmatic adjustments also carry with them normative assumptions about citizenship and modes of governance. Such adjustments thereby urge local actors to conform to these ideological premises about rights, responsibilities, and entitlements. To forge a world more universally governable, development projects employ similar strategies for structural change, expecting to produce similar (and predictably market-friendly) results. Similarly, international donors like the Global Fund want to see the HIV control interventions they trust, interventions proven effective elsewhere, implemented with fidelity in the Ukrainian context. When they mandate specific reporting practices for contractors, Global Fund portfolio managers are not simply interested in seeing deliverable products created by local efforts to extend preventative health care to people who use drugs. They are also interested in seeing legible, predictable results that make sense within their preexisting system of scientific beliefs.

HIV and other infectious diseases associated with injection drug use are examples of what Erin Koch has called "non-profit diseases" (Koch 2013, 17): health concerns that do not attract market attention because the affected population lacks the financial means necessary to establish themselves as a lucrative consumer base. Interestingly, the Global Fund perceives the target population for MAT as individuals who are not only poor but also are typically engaged in petty criminal activity as a direct result of their substance use disorder. In a 2005 interview, Murotboki Beknazarov, a grant implementation unit manager for the Global Fund, suggested that people who use drugs "will be less dangerous to society if they receive free-of-charge doses [of medications used for MAT] daily, they will not be involved in stealing to purchase such doses" ("Interview with the Global Fund" 2005). In other words, not only can people who need MAT not be expected to pay for this form of treatment, they can also be expected to violate social norms (as well as the law) without it. Here lies the challenge, though: the goal of creating self-governing, responsibilized citizens through a transition to market-based health-care systems, which so often lies at the heart of global health interventions (Keshavjee 2014; Nichter 1989; Robins 2006), cannot be met when the target population's interaction with the market economy is, itself, understood to be deviant or pathological. Responsibility for governance, therefore, is shifted to organizations like Better Together that must do the work of bringing health-care systems and health-care users into contact with one another to fulfill the Global Fund's priorities for HIV control.

Though hardly unique to this part of the world, donors' poor understanding of local sociocultural contexts often hinders global health projects in the post-Soviet sphere. Sociologist Alexandra Hrycak characterizes "the encounter between the unexamined assumptions of foreign aid projects and the cultural presuppositions, existing networks, and organizational strategies of local actors" (Hrycak 2006, 70–71) as a common source of difficulty for development projects in Ukraine. Similarly, anthropologist Michelle Rivkin-Fish has attributed historically intractable disagreements between medical professionals in Russia and international health-care development organizations to the foreigners' "[failure to] consider how their own knowledge was shaped by historical, cultural, and institutional experiences that Post-Soviets might not share" (Rivkin-Fish 2005, 2). In short, global health projects have a long history of confronting post-Soviet citizens with unfamiliar notions of citizenship (Zigon 2010), conflicting structures of authority (Mason 2016), and practical goals that simply cannot be met due to financial limitations felt at either the institutional (Koch 2013) or the individual level (Keshavjee 2014). Frustration, therefore, often follows closely behind the expectation that post-Soviet actors—or the statistical measures through which those actors are "captured" and represented—will display certain characteristics of personhood or citizenship that these individuals have not embodied before. In response to these pressures, the Global Fund, Ukrainian authorities, and local organizations like Better Together try to influence one another, each hoping to make the others conform in some way to their preferred way of work. The construction of socioscientific networks is the primary means by which this is accomplished.

French sociologist Michel Callon describes the construction of these networks as a two-stage process: first, *interessement*, "to impose and stabilize the identity of other actors" in relation to a specific problem (Callon 1986, 208), and second, *enrolment*, "the device by which a set of interrelated roles is defined and attributed to actors who accept them" (Callon 1986, 211). For example, I was subject to forces of *interessement* at the MAT clinic in Odessa's TB hospital, when acting physicians tried to teach me how to interpret their patients' personal stories (see chapter 4). In making this effort, the doctors sought to establish me as a professional ally—an actor separated from their patient population through social status and expertise. They encouraged me to see myself, a research professional, as "one of them" by defining me in opposition to their clients. They then sought my *enrolment*, my formal adoption of this social role, by urging my skepticism about their patients' claims to behaviors like abstinence from illicit drugs and matters of routine self-care.

If I could be made a skeptic, and if I could wield that skepticism from a position of professional authority, then the construction of my social identity as a member of their professional class would have been complete. Fortunately, I was able to avoid being clearly situated within the socioscientific networks of MAT clinics by moving freely through the institutions I visited, often positioning myself (both physically and metaphorically) away from those few who sought to use me to their advantage and claim my voice as their own. Nevertheless, the desire—if not the *need*—to make me a legible actor within these networks followed me through my fieldwork from beginning to end.

As the most financially powerful actor working in the realm of harm reduction in Ukraine, the Global Fund must also directly concern itself with the tasks of *interessement* and *enrolment* by working to establish a network of reliable social actors in Ukraine who can faithfully represent their interests and fulfill the promise of evidence-based public health practice. This means recruiting actors—including major organizations like the Alliance and, further down the line, local NGOs like Better Together—to take part in projects of their design and compelling those actors to implement the Global Fund's required protocols with fidelity. The measure of the *interessement* and *enrolment* of local actors into this specific scientific network is in the program indicators that local partners assemble for Global Fund approval. Data reporting, in other words, is not simply good for monitoring program activities. It also lets network actors track how successfully each organization is doing their due diligence by "sticking to the script" as the Global Fund has defined it.

Any success the Global Fund has achieved in compelling Ukrainian actors to conform to the social roles assigned to them (and some success has indeed been achieved) has been gained in spite of long odds: the bureaucratic worlds of post-Soviet business, politics, and work frequently prove to be fundamentally unauditable in the Western sense of the word. This has been true on many a grand scale. Stephen Collier, for example, has detailed painfully futile attempts to privatize public utilities, like water and gas, in cities where early Soviet city planners working within a centralized economy saw no reason to include things like water or gas meters in their designs. The infrastructure that made access to these public utilities possible lacked the very technology necessary to make those utilities "visible" in a way that would allow them to be bought or sold as commodities (2011). This unauditability has also held true on smaller scales, such as the business records of a single

n Poland undergoing privatization in the 1990s. Anthro-
Dunn has described the challenges faced by American
ng for companies like Gerber, Kraft, and Heinz when
ate the market value of the factory. All kinds of uncertain-
Soviet accounting system, which often focused on factory
p...... ncglecting to record the costs or mechanisms of obtaining raw
materials, could only be translated into American accounting systems through
best estimates and outright guesses. Unsurprisingly, different assessments of
the factory's worth varied by millions of dollars (2004).

To date, the most significant challenge faced by the Global Fund in its
attempts to build a socioscientific network has been the *enrolment* of the
Ukrainian government and efforts to compel national leaders to act "ratio-
nally" in the face of a growing HIV epidemic. The MoH and its representative actors have long carried out activities according to their own needs and
convened alternative scientific networks in-line with their own political views
about where people who use drugs belong in the national body politic. In
the Soviet era, the state perceived alcohol and drug use not simply as un-
healthy but, also fundamentally "anti-social" behaviors that tore "correct" social relationships asunder and threatened the entire socialist utopian project
(Starks 2008). Similar views proliferate in popular imagination in Ukraine
today, and many Ukrainian authorities continue to pursue the *enrolment* of
clinics, physicians, and other social actors into the harsh policing of drug-
use behaviors and the abandonment of individuals who use drugs by social
support and health-care infrastructures.

This approach was not wholly inconsistent with Soviet-era politics of compulsory treatment for substance use, which included the dispatching of police to resolve work truancy complaints and the incarceration of individuals
who chronically used drugs in labor camps. These camps were meant to impart corrective habits onto those forced into them but mostly just succeeded
in reproducing their isolation from the rest of society (Raikhel 2016). The
blurring of medical and criminal authority over substance use continues today
through the work of the MoH and local police, both institutional legacies of
their Soviet predecessors. The MoH, therefore, continues to be both directly
and indirectly complicit in strict and unethical policing of people who use
drugs and the programs that serve them. Harm reduction organizations sit
at the juncture of these many agendas, forced to satisfy multiple masters for
the sake of the clients they serve.

Evidence-Based Global Health in Practice

Back in Gennadiy's office, paperwork routinely piled up. Gennadiy empha-sized that a number of these records were essential for the long-term finan-cial management of his organization. How were they to know how many syringes they needed to buy next month, for example, without a record of how many they had distributed the month before? Though keeping things like supply inventories up to date seemed perfectly reasonable things to do, many of their mandated logs and spreadsheets seemed particularly pro forma to both of us—paperwork that needed doing simply for the sake of being done. One such example was a log that tracked not only individual client vis-its but also the specific supplies (the number of condoms or clean socks or new syringes) each client took on a given occasion. The utility of knowing how frequently clients returned for services and how many supplies, in gen-eral were distributed seemed obvious, but the linking of specific supplies to specific clients less so. How the social workers at Better Together were to make use of that information to improve client services was especially un-clear. Gennadiy and I shared the suspicion that those logs were creating rich and interesting data sets that no one at the local or the international level would ever take the time to analyze.

Many of the detailed data collection requirements mandated by the Global Fund reflect this donor agency's commitment to "evidence-based interven-tions that aim to ensure access to HIV prevention, treatment, and care and support for most-at-risk populations" (Global Fund 2010). Evidence-based practice, simply defined, is "the conscientious, explicit, and conscious use of current best evidence in making decisions about the care of individual pa-tients" (Sackett et al. 1996, 71). Evidence-based approaches have been adopted as the "gold standard" of medical decision making by the WHO (2012) and the Global Fund (Global Fund 2012). It is, therefore, a form of knowledge production that functions well in the sociocultural environment of these in-ternational elites.

The Global Fund prioritizes specific programs in its HIV prevention work, such as syringe access and MAT, because a large body of scientific evi-dence indicates that these programs are able to efficiently prevent the spread of HIV among people who are using illicit drugs (Abdul-Quader et al. 2013; Aspinall et al. 2014; Mattick et al. 2009). The fact that such programs *can* work, however, does not necessarily mean that they *will* work if improperly implemented, that they are easy to operate, or that they are foolproof. The need to constantly evaluate program efficacy serves as ample justification (according to this international view) for the detailed accounting the Global Fund requires. The records that Gennadiy and his staff keep, tracking every client, every needle, and every dollar are able to provide donors with the assurance that the program is being run "correctly." They ensure that the *enrolment* of local actors into the Global Fund's socioscientific network has been successful.

There is, in fact, a cascade of auditing activities designed to ensure the *enrolment* of Better Together in this socioscientific network. The Global Fund must, first and foremost, successfully *enrole* its primary grant recipient, the Alliance. The staff of the Alliance must, in turn, successfully *enrole* the staff of NGOs that subcontract through them to provide the services that Global Fund monies support—people like Gennadiy. Recursive auditing practices, in which NGOs report to the Alliance and the Alliance reports to the Global Fund, mandate transparency between organizations, allowing more powerful actors to achieve desired levels of social control; these reporting practices were, in Elizabeth Dunn's words, "set up as a proxy for external governance, because it supposedly forces [organizations] to govern [themselves]" (2004, 41). In a 2010 interview, a program manager at the Alliance confirmed this relationship, explaining her organization's monitoring practices as follows:

> The Global Fund requires us to follow the money and look where it's being spent. Is it going to the program or not? So there's a lot of program monitoring that's connected to this issue. Also there's the financial monitoring which is separate. Like audits—we have an audit which tracks all the spending accounts and books, but as far as programmatic monitoring, we just want to make sure that we are reaching the clients, that there is coverage, and that we know that they are receiving what we are procuring.

For the Alliance, proper *enrolment*, then, is evidenced through visible and auditable documentation of the flow of funds through harm reduction organizations as well as the flow of targeted populations through the programs they offer.

Despite the need to outwardly display proper *enrolment* to their benefactors, local organizations often find gaps or, to use Erin Koch's term, "slippages" (Koch 2013) in these standardized audit practices, which they can exploit for the benefit of their operation. This is because, as medical anthropologist Michelle Parsons has observed, "Rules are not always fixed" (2014, 51), and structures can enable new forms agency by allowing actors the opportunity to maneuver around them. One of the most interesting examples, to my mind, was a documentational work-around that staff at Better Together developed in response to a reporting rule that did not fit their clients' needs. In addition to the one-for-one rule and the ten-syringes-per-person-per-day rule, a third rule allowed Better Together's syringe access program participants to collect syringes for as many as ten other people by presenting all ten client ID cards when they came to the program. Though a seemingly helpful accommodation for those clients who faced difficulty traveling to their office, the impracticalities of this arrangement were numerous. The program still needed to operate on a one-for-one basis, yet rarely did clients picking up supplies for a group have as many as one hundred used syringes to hand over. Most found the idea of carrying giant containers of used syringes filled with *shirka* residue around the streets of Odessa to be patently absurd. Further, Better Together's program ID cards were clients' only recourse if they were harassed by local police, as a city ordinance provided immunity to those registered in Better Together's program from criminal charges for possessing drug paraphernalia. The likelihood that as many as ten participants would willingly surrender that card to someone else for an undetermined period of time was, understandably, negligible.

Though the Global Fund was not necessarily interested in micromanaging the minor details of Better Together's program model, Gennadiy and his staff still needed to produce documentation that reflected their organization's compliance with the Global Fund's standards of practice. However, certain assumptions about how such organizations *would* operate were built into mandated reporting practices, inadvertently allowing the staff of Better Together the statistical wiggle room they needed to modify their program operations without compromising the objective measures reflected in their reporting. For example, the problem of clients' lack of needles to turn in was easily resolved by the fact that there was no space on the mandated reporting forms to record the number of syringes collected for disposal. It was simply assumed that a one-for-one exchange would occur. Thus, the collection of used needles was sufficiently implied by a record of the corresponding number of clean syringes being handed out.

In a slightly more creative twist, Better Together's staff overcame the second problem, the requirement that patients present multiple ID cards, by adapting a technique that had long been a core strategy of business management in the deficit-riddled Soviet economy: they kept two sets of books. Data transmitted to the Global Fund were recorded in binders stuffed thick with standardized forms. In addition to this, staff also kept ancillary records in small spiral notebooks, the likes of which would fit easily into a purse or back pocket. Through detailed, handwritten notes and lists of participant ID numbers, grouped according to which ones "went together," the staff painstakingly detailed the various social networks this program had tapped into and the roles that different individuals played within those networks. It was documented in these small notebooks, for example, that a particular client whom I met during my visit distributes clean injection equipment to her boyfriend, several housemates, and a few of her close friends who have difficulty making the trip. Each of these contacts had been officially registered in the program and assigned an ID number. In one of the program staff's notebooks, these contacts were listed not by name but by ID number below that of the client who served as a de facto secondary distribution point for that social network. Their links to the program—and to each other—were numerically encoded the social worker's curly longhand, allowing staff to record each true client visit in their notebooks while logging what the Global Fund considered to be "complete" information on mandated reporting forms: a client ID written down for every set of ten syringes given out, when in reality eighty or ninety syringes were given out to a single person all at once.

After more than a decade of describing these observations to others, I have found that most people—anthropologists, public health professionals, and even Ukrainians who work outside these public health professions—are strongly inclined to interpret Better Together's double bookkeeping practice as a form of deception. Some even saw it as an act of corruption. Similarly, on countless occasions throughout my research, I heard international elites—especially foreign program directors allied with Western aid or development organizations—describe "nonstandard" local business practices (such as Better Together's double books) as a destructive vestige of the Soviet mentality against which their professions as development experts obliged them to struggle. These complaints mirrored with near perfection the chagrin, described by Dunn, of the accountants for Gerber and Heinz who were tasked with making sense of Soviet-era books from the Polish baby-food factory.

The conclusion that Better Together was up to no good, however, placed emphasis on the presumed self-serving (and, by extension, nefarious) purposes of double bookkeeping, while ignoring the ways in which "honest" or "transparent" accounting practices are also designed to fulfill specific personal or political goals. The Global Fund's mandated accounting practices, for example, may seem straightforward and politically neutral to individuals who are accustomed to such ways of doing business. However, those who are unaccustomed to organizational transparency and automated forms of oversight may find the Global Fund's auditing methods intrusive or even inappropriate. Likewise, locally generated accounting and data recording processes, like the records kept in Better Together's handheld notebooks, served specific, locally meaningful needs that may have appeared unimportant or simply gone unnoticed by their foreign donors. As stated previously, the Global Fund's reporting practices reflect specific management priorities: namely, the appropriate movement of funds through their contractors and subcontractors, and the movement of individuals appropriately targeted by harm reduction efforts through the programs they fund. Thus, a linchpin in the feasibility of Better Together's modified data collection practices is the fact that their "second books" do not directly interfere with the data collection that the Global Fund mandates. Clients are still registered. Syringes are still counted. The personal records kept by the syringe access program staff are additive, an extra act of documentation that benefits the organization but is ultimately of little concern to its donors. The details of clients' social networking are not, for international organizations, a matter of immediate concern. There is no need to *enrole* local NGOs by mandating such records.

It also bears mentioning that the Global Fund's attempts to create disciplined actors within its network are directed at service organizations, such as Better Together, not on the populations they serve. Rather than require payment or self-presentation at the clinic or any other standard features of the responsibilized, neoliberal consumer-subjects that many global health efforts aim to produce, the Global Fund focuses its auditing practices on the appropriate management and provision of *services* for people who use drugs, people whom service organizations like Better Together are, themselves, obliged to identify, link with, and offer care. Thus, the reporting practices that Better Together participates in as a subcontractor for the Global Fund help enforce its own *enrolment* as an entity specially designed to respond to the needs of Ukrainians who use drugs—Ukrainians who constitute a unique counterpublic, which must be classified separately from wider society and afforded their "right to health" in specially tailored ways.

The Enforcement of Other Logics

The ability to navigate the practical and ethical perils of *enrolment* in a socio-scientific network is a skill that clinicians and public health service workers have had to learn, first, to maintain good relations with the Global Fund, and second, to survive in the regulatory environment created by the Ukrainian MoH. The MoH wields a much smaller budget than the Global Fund and must work within the limits of a health-care system that has maintained many of the structures and institutions native to the Soviet-style management of substance use. These include the medical specialization of "narcology" and the view that people who use drugs are particularly dangerous individuals who need to be managed and contained for the protection of wider society. Even as the MoH allows MAT clinics and syringe access programs to operate, the state has long managed these programs in ways meant to contain their potential damage to society at large rather than support the health of the individuals they target. In contrast to the Global Fund's approach, their focus is not so much on policing individual organizations but on policing the individuals whom those organizations serve. In concrete terms, this means clinicians and program directors are subject to state mandates to complete duplicate, triplicate, and sometimes even quadruplicate records of their patients' activities, rendering those patients visible to multiple mechanisms of state surveillance.

The data regimes of the Ukrainian MoH (and of its Soviet predecessor) have historically appeared to hinder rather than help the functioning of health-care systems—at least by Western standards. The Soviet health ministry, for example, regularly accounted for the number of personnel in a hospital and the number of procedures performed, but did not follow indicators of the effectiveness of care (Raikhel 2016). Rivken-Fish has observed the legacy of these rules in contemporary Russia, where money is still budgeted to hospitals according to the number of beds filled, encouraging over-hospitalization and longer stays for those admitted (2005). The Ukrainian MoH does record and fund health-care facilities based on patient outcomes, but this practice has arguably generated a worse effect: the refusal to treat patients who appear to threaten a hospital's record of good outcomes.

Consequently, stories of mistreatment by medical professionals abounded in my interviews with MAT patients. One particularly devastating story, recounted to me by the staff of an outreach organization in the central Ukrainian city of Cherkasy, involved a woman, known to engage in opioid use, who suffered a hemorrhage following a miscarriage. Staff at the local hospital in her catchment area allegedly refused to let her through the front door, knowing that her chances of death were high. If she was going to die anyway, better that she do it outside of the hospital facilities. The woman did eventually receive the care she needed, but only after staff from the outreach organization spent a significant portion of the afternoon working their social connections and pulling strings to have her seen by a qualified professional.

In contrast to these disturbing tales, my experience indicates that physicians who serve patients in MAT clinics are typically motivated by a sense of a calling to this work and understand their full participation in these illogical systems of reporting imposed upon them as an act they must willingly take on for the well-being of their patients. While observing at an MAT clinic in L'viv in 2013, the physician who ran the program, a kind, middle-aged man named Aleksey, patiently walked me through all the paperwork that the MoH obliged him to complete each day. He kept it all arranged in tight, orderly piles across his desk. One form logged the exact dosage of buprenorphine that each client received each day. In his capacity as the lead physician, he had to complete and sign each daily entry. A second form was used to monitor whether the dose indicated on the first form had been delivered to the patient and fully consumed. The nurse on duty and each patient, in turn, must sign this form when the dosing takes place. A third form, again signed by the doctor, logs the time and date that each client arrived at the clinic for medication. "This is in case the police come around asking questions," Aleksey explained. This form served as both an indicator of patients' compliance with the rules of the program and an alibi in case the police accused them of involvement in some kind of trouble around town.

The absurdity of these multiple logging and signing exercises is compounded by the fact that Ukraine has no functional electronic medical record system to speak of. Medical records and monitoring forms are kept on

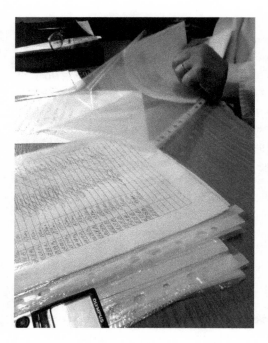

A sample of the many handwritten forms that must be maintained in hard copy at a busy MAT clinic in L'viv. Photo by author.

paper, never scanned, never digitized, never transferrable except in hard copy. It is incredibly difficult to do something as simple as a medical chart review—a post hoc form of medical research wherein data from an array of health records are aggregated and analyzed to study trends in patient outcomes—because it is impossible to generate databases of de-identified health information. All data are kept on physical sheets of paper with every patient's name, date of birth, and contact information printed across the top. In 2012, a colleague of mine from the United States was able to conduct a limited chart review at a regional HIV hospital in L'viv only because the head doctor volunteered to spend several of her afternoons obscuring patient identifiers on medical records with masking tape. She covered the headers of every single paper file needed and then delicately removed the masking strips when the review was complete so the records could be refiled. This effort was nothing short of extraordinary. Similarly, the records Aleksey kept, tracking every detail of his patients' behavior in the clinic, are prohibitively cumbersome to analyze en masse and contain data that are largely useless for measuring a patient's progress through treatment or assessing the efficacy of a particular clinic.

Local police departments, which have historically served as the enforcers of compulsory treatment or incarceration orders for people who chronically use drugs, also serve as the main enforcers of MAT programs and their adherence to the MoH's reporting requirements. As a result, the risks of legal and criminal ramifications for improperly maintained records were very real. Furthermore, local police often have their own interests to consider in the management of people who use drugs. It was common knowledge among my informants (including clinicians, harm reduction staff, and people who use drugs) that the police were in control of the street-level drug market in Ukraine (see chapter 4). Their financial interest in harassing and extorting consumers in that market for profit has been well documented (Human Rights Watch 2006; Mimiaga et al. 2010; Spicer et al. 2011), but my informants emphasized the resentment that many police officers hold for MAT programs in particular. Police allegedly believe these clinics to simultaneously enable drug use by giving away free narcotics *and* steal paying clients away from police officers' own illegal drug-selling operations. Because they stand to lose profits on two fronts (reduced drug sales and reduced opportunities for extortion), police officers have been known to engage in the extrajudicial harassment of MAT providers and patients, often deterring users from seeking services in the first place.

I witnessed the impact of this harassment firsthand while shadowing outreach workers from Better Together in 2007. We were parked on the outskirts of town in a converted minibus that served as a mobile syringe access point, rapid testing facility, and medical consultation site. After backing into the designated parking spot and opening the van doors for business, a steady stream of clients began passing by to collect supplies and see members of the staff. Then, all of a sudden, something changed. I saw eyes darting around, bags hastily thrown over shoulders, and the crowd on the sidewalk evaporate. The street fell into an eerie quiet. Confused, I turned to Katya, the lead outreach worker on this shift, and asked her what had just happened. She pursed her lips and nodded in the direction of two unremarkable-looking men chatting across the street. "Police," she said. "There's no point in sticking around here." And with that, we packed up and returned to the office two hours ahead of schedule.

Physicians working in MAT clinics also endure police harassment and other legal ramifications for allegations of improperly maintained documents and certifications. Local police officers have been known to show up at clinics unannounced and demand to see current paperwork, sometimes taking copies of patients' confidential medical records with them (Golovanevskaya, Vlasenko, and Saucier 2012). Clinicians at MAT clinics are at constant risk not simply because a police officer's word could easily be taken over their own in local courts but also because they are obliged to follow official regulations governing the provision of MAT that clearly contradict one another. One example of such legislation is joint order No. 306/680/21/66/5, ratified by the MoH, the Ministry of Internal Affairs, and the prosecutor's office. This order requires, first, that substance use disorder be diagnosed by a medical committee, and second, that a patient receiving the diagnosis be placed on a national registry of known *narkomany*. When this order was passed, a contradictory piece of legislation was still in effect: MoH order No. 645, which stated that a physician may independently diagnose a patient with substance use disorder and that a patient may only be placed on the national registry if that patient gives permission to do so.

This very legal ambiguity was used in 2010 as a pretext for arresting Yaroslav Olendr, a physician in charge of an MAT clinic in Ternopil'. Dr. Olendr was arrested for his alleged failure to consult with a full medical committee before prescribing methadone to one of his patients and kept under house arrest for several months (Golovanevskaya, Vlasenko, and Saucier 2012). Around the same time, Dr. Ilya Podolyan, who ran an MAT clinic in Odessa, was arrested, along with two of his nurses, during a police raid on his clinic. He was at first released without charges but a month later, rearrested on forty-two separate counts of illegal drug trafficking—an act that he had allegedly committed by distributing to his patients their daily prescriptions of methadone (Cohen 2010; International HIV/AIDS Alliance in Ukraine 2010). The offending act, which rendered his medical practices a criminal enterprise in the eyes of legal authorities, was his failure to inform the MoH of an address change at his clinic in a timely manner (Cohen 2010). Dr. Podolyan's arrest effectively suspended medical service for the approximately two hundred patients receiving MAT at his clinic.

Most Ukrainian clinicians whom I interviewed considered many MoH rules to be deliberately written to be impossible to follow. In addition to the burdensome documentation they must keep, my informants described requirements such as the dedication of a separate room in a hospital or clinic for storing MAT drugs (difficult when physical space is at a premium); mandatory security and alarm systems for the rooms where methadone and buprenorphine are stored (difficult when money is at a premium); and regulations stipulating that MAT drugs must be distributed in a clearly marked and designated location in the clinic (difficult when patient privacy is at a premium). In a 2010 interview, a young staffer at the Alliance named Dima was very clear in his assertion that these rules were deliberately complicated. "They want to create a culture of fear," he told me. "They create rules that no one can possibly follow, so that you are always in violation of something. That way, they can threaten you with consequences anytime you have upset the wrong person." What Dima described is *enrolment* under duress.

To keep these threats at bay, harm reduction organizations must outwardly cede to the desires of the MoH and police forces. Keeping triplicate and quadruplicate forms of their clients' activities is one such capitulation. In contrast to the Global Fund's socioscientific network, the social roles and relations convened by Ukrainian authorities are designed to produce a more intimate form of biopolitical control over individuals who use drugs and the spaces in which they exist. This includes not only the streets and neighborhoods that local police officers patrol but also the clinics and programs specifically designed to serve individuals with a history of substance use. This overzealous monitoring allows MAT clinicians the opportunity to present themselves as willing adherents to the priorities of the MoH and the police, as successfully *enroled* actors in the socioscientific networks established by local authorities. The invasive monitoring of clients ultimately results in sacrifices to the personal freedoms they experience in and around their program offices; however, without such willingness to present themselves as *enroled* in this authoritarian project, these clinics would likely be prevented from operating in the first place.

Chimeric Power

Though audit culture is often seen as a tool of neoliberal power and knowledge, the use of burdensome paperwork to police harm reduction organizations and MAT clinics, and even the budgeting of funds for state hospitals according to beds filled and procedures completed, reveal not only that the exertion of control through audit cultures can be effective *outside* of neoliberal systems but also that this strategy is generated and used in spaces beyond neoliberal influence. Furthermore, these cases illustrate how auditing practices can function through multiple mechanisms of power toward multiple, even contradictory, goals at the same time. In other words, audits can be chimeric instruments of biopower.

Michel Foucault laid the groundwork for contemporary theories of neoliberalism and biopower by distinguishing between power enacted through disciplinary means and power enacted through physical punishment (1977). Discipline is able to exert power over bodies by internalizing mechanisms of governance within the subject. For example, an American citizen might choose to file taxes correctly and pay anything owed as soon as it is due, even without direct governmental oversight, because the constant threat of a random audit by the Internal Revenue Service has made it preferable to always follow the tax law rather than risk being caught in violation. Punishment, on the other hand, has historically functioned as a mechanism of power "that not only did not hesitate to exert itself directly on bodies, but was exalted and strengthened by its manifestations; . . . that presented rules and obligations as personal bonds, a breach of which constituted an offense and called for vengeance; a power for which disobedience was an act of hostility . . . that had to demonstrate not why it enforced its laws but *who were its enemies*" (Foucault 1977, 57; emphasis added). Though Foucault wrote of the evolution of biopower as a gradual transition, with torture- and punishment-based enactments of power gradually giving way to the disciplinary technologies that constitute modern forms of governance, little anthropological theory exists to address these two forms of biopower in stable coexistence with one another. However, adopting a broader view of what might constitute violence in a market economy allows us to do precisely that.

Take the two regimes of data collection that harm reduction programs are obliged to maintain—one endorsed by the Global Fund, the other by the MoH. Each frames people who use drugs as two different kinds of publics: as a counterpublic, a population distinct from mainstream society marked by unique characteristics and requiring its own form of governance and service, or as an antipublic, a collection of criminal outsiders who must be contained for the protection of the general population. These regimes thereby assert different normative assumptions about people who use drugs and the forms of citizenship to which they are entitled, complicating the social careers of these individuals and forcing Ukrainian public health workers to scaffold contradictory forms of governmentality over their clients. Both conform neatly to the tenets of audit culture, compelling harm reduction organizations and MAT clinics to self-govern and conform to reporting requirements on their own. But consider also the consequences of running afoul of these two controlling entities. The local police have quite clearly demonstrated their willingness to imprison doctors on flimsy charges. Similarly, the Global Fund has demonstrated its willingness to rescind the financial resources it provides by removing the MoH as Ukraine's primary grant recipient in 2004.

The withdrawal of program funding is certainly not the same thing as physical intimidation, extortion, or wrongful imprisonment, which the Ukrainian police have allegedly practiced, but it can be viewed as a form of economic violence against those state entities and sectors of civil society reliant on this support. If either the Alliance or the Global Fund decided that Better Together was not a good-faith actor and terminated their agreement, Gennadiy would be out of a job; so would Katya and the rest of the outreach workers they employed. Clients might continue receiving services through a different organization, but social relationships would be severed, trust lost, and vulnerability to police abuse at least temporarily increased. Whether or not the Global Fund intended to make an example of the MoH by withdrawing its financial commitments, it succeeded in doing so, producing its own system of audits supported simultaneously by disciplinary mechanisms and threats of economic punishment.

Just as audit culture is not unique to neoliberalism, it is fair to say that chimeric forms of biopower are not unique to post-Soviet society. The blurring of disciplinary and punitive technologies in American drug courts, extreme military or fraternity hazing rituals, even the street harassment of women immediately come to mind. What this Ukrainian example shows, however, is the ease with which such chimeras of control can emerge around marginalized groups that are perceived as an exception—or a threat against— the body politic of the true public.

Cucumbers and the Politics of Counting Them

In September 2012, I was invited to visit a narcological dispensary in Simferopol, Crimea. Two physicians, Ivan and Pavel, managed this clinic, which served around two hundred patients daily. I met both doctors in Ivan's office where I spent the afternoon discussing the finer points of their work. Over tea and candies, we conversed about Ukrainian politics, the epidemiology of HIV, and the practicalities of patient care in an MAT program.

"The problem here is that we have people who settle into methadone treatment [Rus: *sidet' na metodone*]." Ivan told me. "They don't want to quit taking the drugs. They say 'this program is alright,' and they just stay there. Of course, there are lots of statistics like that, which can make this program look like a failure." This was an ironic statement, because his clinic was clearly not failing. He ran one of the largest MAT clinics in the region, and the level of satisfaction his patients had with their care was remarkably high. He and his partner, Pavel, had even been identified by members of the Global Fund's harm reduction network as a source of best practices for MAT in Ukraine. He went on, "those wouldn't just be statistics for just social outcomes either. It could be the percentage of patients with HIV, the percentage of patients with TB, the percentage who have started treatment for other diseases since they entered this program."

"You know," Pavel interrupted him, "we have this one well-known statistic here. Lots of people like green cucumbers, especially in the summer when they are very fresh. Everybody eats them. We could say that nearly 80 percent of the people in Ukraine eat green cucumbers on any given day in the summer, including the people who die. So that's where we get the well-known statistical fact that 80 percent of people who die in the summer have 'eating cucumbers' listed as their cause of death!" Ivan and Pavel erupted into laughter.

The humor behind Pavel's joke was predicated on the doctors' shared belief that the MoH lacked the political will to respond seriously to Ukraine's very pressing public health problems and support internationally accepted standards of evidence-based practice. That lack of rationality, in their minds, was evident not only in the MoH's failure to maintain quality epidemiological data on the basic state of public health in Ukraine but also in what they saw as the obvious political motivations for the MoH's burdensome record-keeping schemes for MAT clinics. Throughout my research, I found this to be a widely-held view among public health professionals in Ukraine. It exists, in part, due to the belief, generated and solidified into common sense during the Soviet era, that the state has an interest in generating statistics only insofar as the data can be manipulated for the state's political purposes. Historian Tricia Starks has observed that the political nature of medical statistics had been discussed by Soviet physicians as far back as the 1920s during the era of the Soviet Union's New Economic Policy. "Statistics," she notes, "should be regarded in the same way as any political utterance—with circumspection" (2008, 66–67). Statistical quantification wagged the dog of the centralized Soviet economy, and, since all scientific knowledge is socially contingent, it can never be cleanly mapped onto an underlying objective "reality." It can, however, be checked for errors against the priorities of a socioscientific network convened to produce specific kinds of data—data that may not be "true" in an objective sense but that all properly *enroled* actors can agree is "correct" (Mason 2016, 97).

In this chapter, I have argued that the MoH and the Global Fund each convened their own socioscientific networks for scientific knowledge production with distinct political goals in mind. The MoH was interested in monitoring things like the coming and going of MAT patients for the purpose of licensing and controlling individual actors implicated in substance use. Their tactics were motivated by the pure biopolitical directive to isolate and contain those perceived to be socially dangerous "Others." The Global Fund, on the other hand, is concerned with the faithful implementation of evidence-based practices, which are deemed to be the most effective and efficient modes of disease prevention across populations. It was interested in the efficient flow of money, clients, and supplies through local organizations; statistics related to testing, linkage to care, and the appropriate allocation of responsibility for participants' engagement with the medical system. Organizations like Better Together were therefore *enroled* in multiple socioscientific networks, subject to multiple audit cultures, and subject to multiple forms of governance and control.

As the next chapter will show, national and international power structures are not the only sites of ontological entanglement in Ukraine's harm reduction world. Many systems of knowledge about *narkomaniia*—some complimentary, some contradictory—exist inside of the clinic as well. This often leaves patients and clinicians at odds as they both pursue what they perceive to be "best" for those whom the clinic serves, revealing yet another site of contention over who *narkomany* are, what they need, and where they belong in society.

Chapter 3

A Deficit of Desire

If you are traveling through Eastern Europe by train, you will have to book a ticket in one of three different classes on the train. These three types of railroad car have all been around (both literally and figuratively) since the Soviet period. Understanding the distinctions between them is especially important if you are taking an overnight train, as the sleeping arrangements they offer are very different. A limited number of high-speed commuter trains have been accommodating intercity passengers since about 2012 (which, once the mechanical issue that caused them to break down on the tracks and strand hundreds of passengers in the middle of nowhere in the dead of winter was corrected, proved to be very convenient). Most ordinary trains, however, plug along at a top speed of about 30 mph. As a result, a significant proportion of train trips in Ukraine are, by default, overnight journeys.

The premium, first-class car is called *lyuks*. It is pronounced like the last syllable of the English word "deluxe," but with a distinctly Ukrainian swivel on the "u." In these cars, passengers are assigned berths in two-person cabins, which are furnished with a soft, cushioned bench seat along each wall, one facing the direction of travel, the other facing the caboose. At night, these bench seats convert into comfortable beds with quality linens for sleeping. While I was conducting my research, these tickets cost the equivalent of USD 100–150, depending on the length of the trip.

The second-class car, *kupe* (a cognate of the French word "coupé"), also features closed cabins and bench seats that convert into beds. However, these cabins accommodate four passengers, not two. For these two additional riders, bunks are affixed to the wall at about eye level on either side of the cabin. These cabins also come equipped with a stereo speaker built into the wall that plays Ukrainian folk music, which you may or may not be able to switch off depending on the condition of the volume controls in your cabin. These tickets typically sold for USD 20–30 each.

The third-class train cars offer a different kind of experience altogether. These cars, called *platzkart*, offer the same double berths found in the *kupe* cars. However, the "cabins" in *platzkart* are completely open. The cabin doors and at least ten inches of the bench-seat cots have been cut away to make room for an interior pathway that runs down the length of the middle of the car. On the other side of the aisle from the truncated bunks, in the remaining two feet between the footpath and the windows of the train car, two narrower bunks are affixed lengthwise against the train's exterior wall, allowing for a total of six people to be stowed in the space typically allotted to a single cabin. Personal privacy in *platzkart* is virtually nonexistent, and one rarely dares walk down the aisle at night, least of all to the treacherous toilet, for fear of ocular injury from the protruding feet of sleeping passengers. For this style of overnight accommodation, the cost of a ticket was typically about USD 8—a significant savings compared to the first- and second-class options.

Platzkart cars are noisy and crowded. Before passengers quiet down for the night—if they quiet down at all—*platzkart* is a scene of much eating, drinking, and merrymaking. Some Ukrainians consume food on trains the way Americans do in movie theaters—which is to say, constantly, but with more alcohol (see Wanner 2010, 4). On one occasion, I was traveling in *platzkart* from Kyiv to Minsk with an American boyfriend. We shared a sleeping area with another man and his wife—we on the berths above, they below. The husband perceived this matter of distributing food on trains to be a very serious one—so much so that he stood up in the middle of the night as we were passing through the fields outside of Homel' and began making a terrible scene. Equally driven by moral dilemma, generosity, and vodka, he admonished himself for failing to properly orient the poor foreigners to Ukrainian culture. *"Gospodi! Ia im ne obiasnil chto takoe poezdnoi uzhin!"* (Dear God! I never told them about train supper!) He then began shaking my startled boyfriend awake and gently but insistently smacking him in the face with sausages and baked apples.

Perhaps this was the sort of insult to my dignity the cashier at the train station in Kyiv envisioned, years later, when I told her my preferred seat assignment on a train to Odessa. Or perhaps she feared something worse. It was not unheard of for wallets to disappear, for women to be harassed, for foreigners to be taken advantage of by passengers with less diplomatic intentions than the fellow with the baked apples. On this particular day, I was standing at her window in the central train station making plans to travel to Odessa with Sergey, a public health advocate I had met only two days earlier. He was a program consultant who advised MAT clinics across Ukraine, helping them to improve their client services and program management skills. He was making site visits to several organizations in the southern regions of Ukraine and invited me to accompany him on his trip. He had already purchased his own tickets by the time we were introduced, so he gave me his seat number and asked me to reserve a space—any available space— in the same car. When I relayed these instructions to the cashier at the ticket booth in Kyiv, she pulled up Sergey's reservation, and her eyes widened. She then pursed her lips and furrowed her brow with palpable discontent. *"Devushka,"* she said. *"Eto . . . platzkart."* (Miss. This is in *platzkart*.)

Despite my best efforts, I was unable to assure her of my familiarity with the Ukrainian rail system, that the foreign woman in front of her had been riding *platzkart* for nearly eight years, and that this option could not strike fear into my heart. "You are a woman traveling apart from your companion," she said. "It's no good. Lots of no-good people there. Tell him to change his ticket so that you can both be in *kupe*." I nominally agreed to do as she said, largely for the sake of ending this conversation, but I insisted on booking the ticket I had already requested. After all, I was still planning to use it. I told her I would have my friend change both of our tickets together when we arrived at the station for our trip the next day.

The cashier saw my ruse. Rather than relieving her concerns, my statements simply reinvigorated her insistence that *platzkart* was no place for a woman like me to be. She appealed to my emotions, to my fear, to my pride.

She didn't just want me to heed her advice. She wanted me to really *want* a different ticket. I understood perfectly well what she needed to be satisfied: a sincere, believable statement that I was abandoning this *platzkart* idea for good. Unfortunately for both of us, I am a terrible liar. In the end, she shook her head and sighed with resignation as I walked away from the counter with my third-class ticket in hand. God help that American woman, she must have thought. There's no telling what trouble she'll fall into.

This chapter is about wanting. It is about the kinds of desire that someone may or may not feel in any meaningful sense but that they are, in one moment or another, obligated to display—the same kind of desire that the cashier selling train tickets hoped I would externalize at her behest. Much like an American child who is taught to smile wide and say "thank you!" when opening a gift they do not want, Ukrainians are often obliged to engage in the praxis of desire as is mandated by their social situation. It is often thought, for example, that a person must truly desire a particular outcome in order to make that outcome manifest. Barren mothers must *want* to have children. Bullied children must *want* to be resilient and strong. Young women boarding trains must *want* to protect their dignity against the denizens of *platzkart*. Otherwise, their indifference will be their downfall. Similarly, I was frequently told throughout my research that people in MAT programs must truly *want* to "get better," otherwise they would never achieve true success in defeating their "addiction."

In this chapter, I describe the narratives of desire that were produced in MAT clinics and reproduced by MAT clinicians and patients in their conversations with me. As Nikolas Rose has observed, "The role of biomedical authority here is not to encourage the passive and compliant patienthood of a previous form of medical citizenship. Citizenship is to be active" (Rose 2007, 143). In these clinics, an "active" social citizen is one who *actively desires* to regain his or her health. Here, I consider the ways in which appeals to the presence or absence of different forms of "desire" fit into local understandings of the social and psychological mechanisms of "addiction" that circulated in and beyond these clinical spaces. I map out a model of "addiction" that is popular among the medical professionals operating Ukraine's MAT programs and the individual prognoses that are contingent on that model. In these moments, we see the "addiction imaginary" seeping through the cracks in professional biomedical discourse. It fills in the gaps in clinical definitions of substance use disorder whenever standardized symptomatologies lack the richness and depth of real human experience. Put another way, when social understandings of "addictive" behaviors do not line up with contemporary theories of individual will, a model of "addiction"—of what it is and what it does—that tackles this incommensurability head-on must be produced.

This is, in fact, the very premise of the "addiction imaginary" concept: notions of "addiction" do not automatically follow the emergence or evolution of substance use behaviors. Rather, "addiction," as an individual state, only appears in a culture's ethopolitical repertoire when abstract theories of individual will and concrete observations of consciousness-altering substance use behaviors appear to be incompatible. Culturally constructed notions of "addiction" (i.e., "addiction imaginaries") must be generated to resolve the philosophical quandaries that substance use behaviors have raised. In their capacity as medical professionals, the clinicians who work in MAT and other harm reduction programs understand quite well how opioids affect the body and the brain. In their capacity as social beings, however, they gravitate, as all people do, toward personal, relatable, narrative understandings of what their patients are going through. Thus, even in the standardized world of the clinical, the culturally determined content of *narkomaniia* in contemporary Ukraine can be discerned.

Soviet Legacies in Contemporary Drug Treatment

In the early Soviet period, two theories of "addiction" fought for prominence among medical professionals. Both theories understood "addictive" behaviors as mediated by a person's relationship with the external environment, but one focused on the social exterior and the other on the psychological interior of the drug-dependent patient. The first of these, which I refer to as the "social etiology of addiction," aligned with the foundational principles of Soviet medicine as established at the First All-Russian Congress of Medical-Sanitary Sections in June 1918. At that time, leaders in the Soviet medical field were especially concerned with "the influence of the economic and social conditions of life on the health of the population and on the means to improve that health" (Solomon 1989, 255). It was thus decided that the medical system would achieve disease prevention through appropriate social and sanitary measures. This social orientation dovetailed with the broader po-

litical view that the Bolshevik Revolution "[had] eliminated the basic antagonistic contradictions between the socioeconomic structure and the health of
the people, and thus did away with the basic source of illness for the workers"
(Field 1967, 39). Under this rubric, drug use behaviors were not characterized as the result of individual failings or moral weakness. Rather, they
were believed to arise, as all diseases did, as a direct result of the destructive
social and economic realities of capitalism.

Interestingly, this thinking led to the brief operation of a methadone-based
MAT program in Leningrad in the 1930s. A physician named Kantorovich
offered this therapy on an experimental basis, taking in allegedly "incurable"
opioid-dependent patients whom he believed still displayed the potential to
become productive members of society again (Latypov 2011, 11). Kantorovich claimed that nearly 70 percent of the patients enrolled in this program
achieved "good" or "satisfactory" results, as measured by the patient's maintenance of family relationships and stability of employment, a claim that flew
in the face of the contemporary view (based on the same logic) that people
with chronic opioid use disorder who continued their drug use even under
the liberating conditions of communism did, in fact, suffer from a "moral
disability," that they were "lacking will" and were therefore useless to both
country and society (Latypov 2011, 11).

This "social etiology" ultimately fell out of favor and was succeeded by
Pavlovian theories rooted in the concept of the conditional reflex. Psychologist Ivan Pavlov defined the conditional reflex as an automatic response to
external stimuli that becomes physically hardwired in the brain through neurological analysis and synthesis of that stimuli (Chilingaryan 1999). Though
this focus on individual physiology appears to depart from the social etiology of human disease derived from Bolshevik politics, it nevertheless succeeded in articulating a concrete link between the environment and specific
pathologies where the explanatory powers of purely social theories failed. For
example, in 1925, Soviet psychologist Mark Sereisky used Pavlov's ideas to
argue that most people who use drugs possess predisposing factors—a "pre-
narcotic personality"—and simply needed a trigger, such as a first dose of
morphine, to awaken the "addictive reflex," the psychological "hook" that
drives compulsive behavior (Latypov 2011, 7). These theories led Soviet clinicians to suspect that if certain stimuli can trigger addictive behaviors, then
different, therapeutically controlled stimuli might be able to repress or elim-
inate them.

A particularly striking example of such a therapeutic approach is "coding" (Rus: *kodirovannie*). This term applies to a variety of therapeutic services, each of which constitutes an attempt to physically rewire a patient's brain by exposing that patient to substance use-discouraging physical and psychological stimuli of various kinds. These practices, typically carried out by a physician, include the delivery of antagonistic pharmaceuticals, clinical performances about the dangers of drinking alcohol or taking drugs while in treatment, and even deliberate deception and chicanery in the health-care setting (Murney 2009; Raikhel 2010). Though this treatment appears to many Ukrainians as a form of charlatanism, many others nevertheless continue to place faith in this procedure and are able to point to family members for whom "coding therapy" has proved to be of enormous help.

Eugene Raikhel's ethnographic research on coding therapy for alcohol addiction in Russia demonstrates that, above all, a patient's *motivation* for sobriety (which is different than their *will* to stay sober) largely determines the success of coding treatment (Raikhel 2010). Raikhel argues that the fear- or aversion-based techniques meant to steer a patient's behavior away from alcohol consumption acts as a sort of "prosthesis of the will, [which allows] for a change in behavior without a change in the self" (Raikhel 2013, 190). Many of the most successful coding patients, those who have been able to abstain from alcohol entirely, return to their clinician regularly to renew their exposure to the drugs or clinical processes that avert their desire to consume, using treatment protocols as "pragmatic aids for the care of the self that bolster the motivations for sobriety" (Raikhel 2013, 210). Thus, coding "works" as a treatment for alcoholism not because external stimuli alone reshape behavior; rather, the desire of the patient to seek out such stimuli and, in doing so, accept the clinicians will as a "prosthesis" or replacement of their own, reshapes their own reflexes and is seen as the primary mechanism of recovery.

The notion that substance use stems from pathological disorders of the will exists far beyond the borders of Ukraine. Historian Marianna Valverde has painstakingly documented this idea in Western cultures across generations, arguing that the dominant twentieth-century view of "addiction" is fundamentally rooted in the idea of a disease of, or deficiency of, the will (1998). She further observes that "scholarly literature on alcoholism and addiction . . . tends to repeat [an] ahistorical and ethnocentric perspective" (1998, 18), and thereby repeats this trope of a troubled will again and again.

Consider, for example, the words of Asa Hutchinson, who was serving as the head of the U.S. Drug Enforcement Agency as he wrote this:

> Drug users become slaves to their habits. They are no longer able to contribute to the community. They do not have healthy relationships with their families. They are no longer able to use their full potential to create ideas or to energetically contribute to society, which is the genius of democracy. They are weakened by the mind-numbing effects of drugs. The entire soul of our society is weakened and our democracy is diminished by drug use. (Hutchinson 2002)

In the large slice of American culture that Hutchinson's views represent, drug use is perceived not as a potentially self-making or social-network-mediating activity, as described in chapter 1, but as a *de*-humanizing, isolating practice that destroys one's sense of self. Linguistic anthropologist Summerson Carr has observed this very logic at work in American talk-therapy programs for people who use drugs, where treatment modalities are intended to recover patients' "true selves," which are believed to be buried underneath thick, impenetrable layers of anger and denial (2010).

Both this popular American view and the Soviet/Pavlovian view of "addiction" have placed the originating pathology of people who use drugs in the realm of individual will. The similarities largely end here, however. The dominant American view of "addiction" is motivated by spiritual, emotional, metaphorical modes of thought. The image of one's "true self" buried under a layer of denial is certainly visually evocative, but it is impossible to say what this could even mean in a biological or clinical sense. The Pavlovian view, by contrast, very clearly translates the development of habits and behaviors into physiological terms. The "free will" of the substance using individual declines, according to this view, because competing habits have become so "hardwired" in the brain that thinking or acting outside of those habits becomes an increasingly difficult task to accomplish. The differences between these two "addiction imaginaries" are rooted, therefore, in how each culture understands individual will to operate. Therefore, Soviet responses to substance use (such as coding, incarceration, and forced labor camps) arguably tell us more about how Soviet culture perceived the nature of human will than it does about the psychology or biology of "addiction." Further, "addiction imaginaries" that perceive MAT to be a useful intervention for opioid use disorder will equally illuminate theories of the will and of the mind belonging to the cultures in which they have developed.

Given all this, it is unsurprising that MAT programs in contemporary Ukraine are sites where new interpretations of drug use and treatment are forged: interpretations that embrace the will of the patients as a necessary element for medical success. Many clinicians perceive "addiction" to be a context-dependent battle between the conscious desires of the "addict" and the drug-seeking behaviors they display. MAT is interpreted, in turn, as a tool with the capacity to intervene in this conflict. Each patient's personal battle is one that, with the right support and scaffolding, can be won if the patient possesses a conscious desire to win it. It is a battle, however, that *can't* be won *without* this conscious desire. This makes the success or failure of MAT as an intervention a direct measure of the strength and appropriateness of a patient's individual will—of how sincerely the person *wants* to be healthy.

What the Patient Wants

There are two ways to discuss "wanting" in Ukraine. The first is a verb: *khotet'* in the Russian language and *khotyty* in Ukrainian. These verbs, very simply, mean "to want." One can use them to indicate very straightforward desires such as "I want to become a teacher" or "I want milk in my coffee." Wanting can also be discussed with a noun: *zhelanie* in Russian, *bazhannia* in Ukrainian. *Zhelanie/bazhannia* can be translated as "desire" or "wanting" or "longing" or "will." It lends itself to the same kind of poetic license in these languages as it does in English. For example, in Russian, you can ascribe to someone *zhelanie umerit'*, a death wish. It is possible to *goret' zhelaniem*, to burn with desire. The distinction between the meanings of these two words is important. While it is possible to want (Rus: *khotet'* / Ukr: *khotyty*) or not want (Rus: *ne khotet'* / Ukr: *ne khotyty*) something without great moral consequence, desire or will (Rus: *zhelanie* / Ukr: *bazhannia*) is a much more fundamental human characteristic. To declare that a person who uses drugs does or does not have the desire to be treated is to assert that someone is either a driven, morally active person or a passive, indifferent, emotionally disengaged individual who is beyond professional help.

On the other end of this emotional spectrum, the concept of "indifference" (Ukr: *baiduzhist'* / Rus: *ravnodushie*) represents the absence of socially appro-

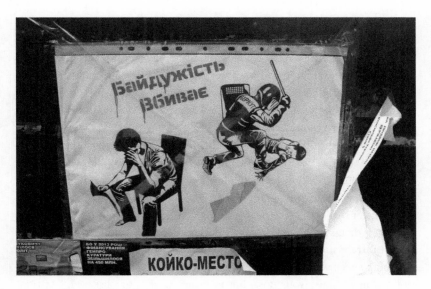

A flier posted in the EuroMaidan protest camp, which reads "Indifference kills"
(Ukr: *Baiduzhist' vbyvaie*). Photo by author.

priate "wanting." It is, in fact, considered to be a social ill in its own right. For example, when I would casually complain to my friends about various difficulties I had encountered throughout my day, they would diligently assign blame to the indifference of others. The cashier at the post office was indifferent to the fact that I needed help buying postage for my parcel. The owner of the BMW who parked across the sidewalk in front of my building was indifferent to the needs of pedestrians. The huffy responses I received from the cashier at the train station who wanted me to move out of *platzkart* can also be explained with an appeal to indifference—not hers, but my own. She was terribly frustrated by my lack of desire to improve my situation. She surely believed I was destructively indifferent to my own well-being.

The visible behaviors of people who use drugs in Ukraine are frequently attributed to pathological levels of indifference or, often, the lack of any desires, even self-serving ones. Subsequently, the active cultivation of desire is generally perceived to be the core therapeutic strategy engaged by MAT clinicians. These ideas were well-illustrated by the case of Timur, a young man in his mid-thirties whom I met in his MAT clinic in L'viv. Timir had been a patient at this clinic for a long time. The care he received was steady, but the details of his treatment were always in flux. He had a hard time settling his body into the physical routine of methadone. When he first began receiving MAT at the AIDS center in his hometown, Timur was given 40 mg of methadone per day. Soon after, he started feeling badly, and his doctor agreed to increase his dose. As they worked to manage his symptoms, Timur's dose crept up, bit by bit, until he reached 150 mg, the upper limit of what his doctor is allowed to prescribe.

When I met him, Timur had already been receiving 150 mg of daily methadone for some time. He complained of body pains, trouble sleeping, and frequent fevers. "My dose [of methadone] right now—it's not enough," he told me. "It doesn't hold me up anymore." The severity of his discomfort motivated him to seek out new strategies for relief. He began by supplementing his MAT drugs with *shirka* from the street. When this stopped working, he began purchasing tramadol from a local pharmacy. He took some each evening to keep withdrawal symptoms from sneaking back in. "Obviously the point is not to raise your dose, but to lower it," Timur observed. "At these levels, I'm worried about my liver." Timur firmly insisted, on multiple occasions, that he genuinely wanted to quit, but the drugs, he said, had too strong a hold on his body.

During a long stay in L'viv in the fall of 2013, I had the opportunity to discuss Timur's situation with his doctor, Alexey. Though this was never overtly confirmed, I was given the impression that Alexey was at least strongly suspicious of, if not quite aware of, Timur's extracurricular drug use. It was also made clear to me that Timur's actions—his ardent refusal to decrease his dose and his unwillingness to comply with the MAT program's prohibitions against the use of illicit drugs—fell squarely into the discursive realm of *zhelanie/bazhannia*. Timur had been told how to treat his "addiction." He had been given the tools that he needs to do so. Yet his problematic drug use persisted. The problem, Alexey said, was not that Timur was physically incapable of quitting. Instead, Timur was too ambivalent—too indifferent—to progress through his treatment. Timur, Alexey told me, suffers from a lack of desire. In fact, Timur could not even be described as *baiduzhii*, or indifferent, because this would indicate a lack of socially appropriate desire—a lack of desire for justice and well-being in the community. One can be *baiduzhii* and still maintain immoral or self-serving desires. Timur, however, stood accused of having no desires at all.

Nearly every clinician I have met in Ukraine, whether or not they have worked directly with MAT programs, has confessed frustration with the absence of any conscious desire to change in some or all of their patients who use drugs. This frustration was especially common among those with specialties outside the realm of substance use disorder. The head doctor of an HIV clinic near Kyiv once threw up his hands in exasperation when I asked about HIV-related deaths among patients with a history of injection drug use. "These deaths," he said, "are related to the anti-social element. They drove themselves straight into their graves. They had no desire to live!" A nurse in a Kyiv TB hospital voiced a similar complaint. As I sat in her office, she scowled at a group of men milling in the entryway outside her department. "Doctors tell them to come here [to this office to receive anti-TB pills]," she said, "but they just hang out, they talk in the hallway, and then they leave. They are alcoholics, 'addicts' [Rus: *alkogoliki, narkomany*]. They have no desire [Rus: *u nikh net zhelaniia*]. Maybe the wife already died, the daughter is already sick. It's all the same to them. They need narcotics to deal with their psychological problems. That's addiction [Rus: *narkomaniia*]."

Those who worked directly with MAT patients perceived the same pattern among their patients; however, I found these clinicians to be much more delicate in their interpretation of each individual case. For example, the director of an outreach program in Mykolaiv, a man who had been passionately advocating for the expansion of MAT in his region since it first became available in 2006, explained to me that different levels of personal desire result in different "kinds" of people who use drugs:

It is important to understand that there are three kinds of "addicts" [*narkomany*]. First, there are those who used street drugs, but managed to fully substitute those street drugs with methadone. They slowly lowered their dose, and eventually quit. But remember, even after they quit, they are still addicts. There is no such thing as a former "addict" [Rus: *byvshikh narkomanov ne byvaiut*]. Second, there are those who don't even think about quitting. They like to keep their methadone regimen at the maximum dose—maybe 150 mg— rather than working to slowly decrease it. They may *want* to quit, but they are too afraid—afraid that they will return to narcotics on the street and completely relapse. The last group is those who never think about quitting methadone and never plan on quitting street drugs either. They continue to use whatever they want the whole time they are on methadone—things like *shirka*.

Many other clinicians explained substance use disorder to me through similar taxonomies of disease. Through these distinctions, an individual's will became a quasi-diagnostic tool for determining the severity of a patient's condition. If you have this desire, you will get better; if you don't, you won't. The ability of MAT programs to affect change in their patients is, therefore, largely determined by a given patient's level of desire to be helped. A strong desire to heal can turn up the dial of treatment efficacy, helping MAT to carry a patient to social and clinical success. MAT, then, is not exactly a "prosthesis of the will," as Eugene Raikhel has described in regard to coding therapy for alcoholism (Raikhel 2013). Rather, MAT is perceived to function, in some ways, as an *extension* of the individual will, a way to develop and grow the "seed" of will that clinicians have sought to impart to each of their patients.

This specific, desire-based etiology of substance use disorder that appears in Ukrainian clinics is a radical departure from the perspectives on addiction and MAT held by the international community. According to these more broadly accepted models, MAT does not produce its therapeutic effect by engaging individual desires. Rather, it works by shutting desires off (WHO 2004a). This dominant view holds that MAT works by "'block[ing]' the euphoric effects of heroin (see chapter 1), thereby discouraging illicit use and thereby relieving the user of the need or desire to seek heroin" (Mattick et al. 2009). By blocking euphoria and simplifying the logistics of staving off withdrawal symptoms, MAT, in this view, frames people who use drugs as fundamentally rational actors and aims to alter their behavior through the rebalancing of factors that affect their decision-making processes. Each patient's internal desires are relevant only insofar as the desire to use drugs is successfully modulated by the intervention, rather than the intervention being modulated by desire.

Instead of reproducing this internationally accepted discourse with fidelity to its core principles, Ukrainian clinicians have integrated the clinical logics and practices of MAT into the local "addiction imaginary." Many clinicians, for example, have made especially strong claims about their expertise on the clinical management of "addiction" based on their alleged familiarity with the lack of desire and will in their patients. They have spent enough time with such patients, these claims go, to identify these features when they are present and note their absence when they are not. For me to gain a better understanding of just how important desire really is, I was often told, I would also have to learn to read these signs—to see as they did past the words and behaviors of their patients into the motivations that drive them. This would help me see what "addiction" truly is and what MAT can do about it.

The Interpretation of Wanting

My first practical lesson in "reading" a patient's desire came from Sergey while we were on one of our voyages through southern Ukraine. As we were traveling together, he introduced me to numerous clinicians and NGO leaders and provided me with an informed perspective on how these different medical and social services interact with each other. We visited a total of eight MAT sites in four different regions, including what was then the Autonomous Republic of Crimea. Our first journey, the one I booked through the incredulous cashier, was to Odessa, was when we paid several visits to Alexandra Nikolaeva's MAT clinic in the central TB hospital.

On our first day there, at Alexandra's request, Sergey and I purchased cheap surgical masks to protect vulnerable patients in the hospitals from any infections we may have brought with us. We strolled down the street across from the hospital gates and entered a little basement pharmacy on the corner. In typical Ukrainian pharmacies, products are kept behind the counter, requiring one to talk to a pharmacist before assessing their inventory and deciding what to buy. As we took our place in line and waited our turn with the pharmacist at the window, the woman at the front of the line completed her purchase and walked passed us toward the door. Her fists were clenched tightly around her newly acquired goods. Sergey turned to me and whispered, "It makes me so sad to see that. She is buying needles and eyedrops." When I expressed confusion about the eye drops, he explained, "It was tropicamide. This is common here. They will drink it, or sometimes inject it. I don't know what it is supposed to do, but lots of people use it."

Tropicamide is an anticholinergic eyedrop. It is most commonly used to dilate pupils during eye exams. This drug was never intended for use by injection. Therefore, no medical research has been carried out on the effects or consequences of consuming tropicamide in this way. Anecdotal evidence collected from social workers and MAT patients during the course of my research supports the conclusion that tropicamide is a mild hallucinogen that amplifies or modulates the effects of opioids. The drops themselves are not very expensive and require no prescription to buy. They are quite accessible to anyone who wants them.

Once Sergey and I had acquired masks at the pharmacy, we turned around and hurried back across the street to the hospital. Alexandra accepted us graciously. Sergey greeted the entire staff with affection. I was properly introduced and allowed to pet half a dozen or so feral cats that were napping in her office. The first order of business was small talk over a generous offering of tea and cookies. After appetites, social and gastronomical, had been sated, Sergey conducted the necessary business of his official site visit, which included a brief survey with the doctors and an inventory check. I munched on a walnut cookie and sat back to observe the clinic in motion.

The first patient we encountered during our stay was a young woman. She had been lingering in the clinic's hallway drinking coffee with a nurse while Sergey and I chatted with the psychologist. Intrigued by our presence, she let herself into the doctor's office to see who we were. As she strode confidently through the door, I immediately recognized her as the woman we had just seen in the pharmacy buying tropicamide. Her name, I soon learned, was Lyuda. At the time of our first meeting, she had only been part of the program for a year and a half—not very long compared to some of the other patients there. She agreed to a formal interview, and took it as an opportunity to share some of her frustrations with the program.

L: Do I like [MAT]? No. At the beginning, when I first came here, I thought it would solve all my problems. Like, I didn't have to hunt for money, didn't have to find drugs on the street. I just came here, took my pills, and went about my business. But after a while . . . well, I can't go anywhere. Not even on weekends, just to visit anyone. It doesn't even matter where. I can't. Because every morning, even on New Years Day, January 1, everyone else is asleep, and I, like a fool—forgive me—I get up and I come here. So, at the beginning it's nice, but it's this vicious circle. And I can't quit. I can't go without this [methadone] . . . psychologically it's very hard.

JC: And how did you come to the decision to start this treatment in the first place?

L: I had a baby. I can't tell you if I am a good mom or a bad mom, but I try. And I do this in order to spend time with her— nearly all my time, not counting the two hours I spend coming here every day. I joined this program so that I could be with her.

Interestingly, through these comments, Lyuda displayed the characteristics of two different "types" of *narkomany*—according to the taxonomy described to me by the social worker in Mykolaiv. On the one hand, she articulated her decision making in a way that highlighted the prioritization of her motherly duties and her will to fulfill them. She needs to spend time with her daughter, so she has taken steps to reduce the portion of her day that she spends acquiring narcotics by switching over to a quicker and more reliable source: MAT. Her decision to begin treatment constituted a practical strategy for managing her multiple priorities: she sacrificed the attention she gave to one (her substance use) so that she could afford greater attention to another (her daughter). The disparaging assessment of the TB nurse, who insisted that *narkomany* "have no will. . . . It's all the same to them [because] that's addiction [Rus: *narkomaniia*]" does not describe Lyuda well. By prioritizing her duties to her child over some of the immediate necessities of her substance use, Lyuda is testifying to her desire to be socially responsible—the very desire that clinicians say their patients need in order to recover.

On the other hand, Lyuda is also strategically controlling the effects of MAT on her body. By adding tropicamide (and perhaps other substances) to her regimen, she is taking steps to alter, adjust, or amplify how she feels on methadone. In her doctor's eyes, her attachment to the physiological effects of opioids—even when her regimen is strictly controlled—is obvious in the actions she takes to modulate and maintain them. This is part of the risk of getting caught using other drugs: not only could she lose privileges in the program or the trust of her clinicians, she would also be saddled with the social stigma of someone unwilling to bear the physical effects of decreasing her opioid use with methadone. She would have to face the consequences of being labeled an "indifferent" patient, a judgment that could have consequences regarding her perceived value as a person and her fitness as a mother.

Lyuda voiced skepticism about MAT as a mechanism for treating her substance use disorder and subsequently ending her drug use all together. She clearly articulated her opinion that the *desire* to quit was not sufficient for overcoming her habits, regardless of how strong or deeply held that desire may be:

JC: How would you describe, in your own words, the goals of this program?

L: To lower . . . I mean, the program gives people . . . we try to live like normal, healthy people. But the truth is that we don't always succeed. Because the brain of an "addict" [Rus: *nar-koman*] is always searching for a high, and here there's no high [Rus: *net kaifa*]. Here it's just, like, I take my pills and I feel fine. Nothing hurts, I sleep regularly, I eat regularly, and everything's fine. And the whole time your dose is decreasing down to that minimum and then you're already going without and we live like normal people. But the reality is that this takes a really long time. A year. Two. It depends on the person. I've already been here for a year and a half and I'm not ready to give it up.

JC: What is it, then, that you would like to gain for yourself?

L: For myself? Honestly? I'd like to wake up in the morning and know that I'm healthy. But that morning won't be coming anytime soon. Because every morning I wake up with just one thought on my mind: I need to get dressed and head out for this place . . . but I'm really tired of it.

JC: If you felt able to, would you want to quit taking methadone entirely?

L: I want to, but I'm not psychologically ready for it. I just know that if I go off the methadone, maybe a week will go by, not more, and I'll start looking for street drugs again. Cause, here [pointing to her chest], it's not just physical, here [pointing again to her chest] it's more important than you could even think.

JC: What do you mean by "ready" to quit? What does "ready" mean?

L: Ready to quit and live like normal people. I can't say that I'm ready because I'm still craving the next high all the time . . . in my head. I struggle with it. I have this daughter who is growing up so fast, and I am very well aware that I need to stop, but it hasn't happened for me.

Lyuda was the first person I heard speak about feeling "stuck" in treatment, unable to change or to quit, but she was far from the last. Understanding the "addiction imaginary" possessed by people who use drugs was one of the primary goals of my research, so I always inquired about the treatment plans they had designed for themselves. My questions were met with a constant refrain of "I want to quit, but I'm just not ready." The significance of this simple phrase was reiterated each time a new person uttered it.

What struck me about this particular moment at the clinic in Odessa, and what Sergey made efforts to drive home to me as we left the clinic that day, was the conflict that Lyuda, the loving mother who topped off her methadone with tropicamide, presented to her medical providers. Both Sergey and Lyuda's psychologist attempted to coach my interpretation of this encounter, telling me that Lyuda will not be successful in her efforts to maintain control over her competing familial and chemical obligations. They especially encouraged me to see that Lyuda was deceiving herself. "You know she's lying to herself, right?" Sergey asked. She may have talked about her daughter and claimed that she wants to live peacefully with her family, but, in the estimation of the medical professionals around her, this was a far cry from reality. She would never be able to quit using drugs until she *really wanted to*, and her tropicamide use was evidence that she didn't really want to. She was not letting herself be treated. She remained indifferent. She was just as "addicted" then, one and a half years into the MAT program, as she was on her first day.

The Metaphysics of Addiction

Many months into our acquaintance, Sergey and I found ourselves sitting across his kitchen table in Kyiv's Osokorky district, eating linden flower honey straight out of the jar with a spoon and once again discussing his work experiences and our beliefs about "addiction." Sergey quietly pondered my questions about what makes MAT successful for some and not for others. I had asked him these questions dozens of times and, by then, they had become almost rhetorical—part of our regular exercise of thinking through what he believed drug-using patients were really up to in these programs. "Of course you have to have the desire to change your behavior," he said, switching from Russian to English, which he often did to emphasize a point. He continued: "*Narkomany*, they must have this desire to quit, because the behavior is bad. But the sin—the consequence—of this behavior is that it destroys your constitution—the thing inside of you that should be the strongest. So, when you are addicted, you understand. You know what is happening to you. But you can do nothing about it." "Addiction," he carefully explained, is characterized by the inability to act upon one's inner desires. You want to quit, but you have lost the self-control needed to do so. He described each person's psyche as a three-part structure: a mind, a body, and a metaphysical connection between the two. When we are sober, all three elements are strong and intact. When we use drugs or alcohol, one or more of them becomes compromised.

He also explained that clinical professionals are able to intervene upon this troubling situation by generating and then capturing the desire of a patient. It is that very desire, in fact, that many treatment professionals hope their efforts will have an effect on. As Sergey explained:

> If someone is seeking rehabilitation with a psychologist, their success will depend on their motivation. They must want to change. The psychologist cannot do all of the work. But the patient cannot get better without the help of the psychologist. Sometimes the patient is motivated inside and just needs to find help. Other times, the psychologist must be skilled at generating their interest, building their desire, lighting a fire in you to change your ways.

When people are engaged in drug use, he argued, their mind, their will, loses its ability to control their actions and behaviors the way they want it to. As they become more and more dependent, people are able to see themselves losing control. They may even retain their desire to be in control, to live their lives, to maintain their relationships, but they are unable to do so. This is why both professional treatment *and* the desire to be treated are necessary for overcoming addiction.

After hearing Sergey and other clinical professionals map out the psychological and emotional terrain of "addiction" in this way, I began seeing echoes of these ideas in my interviews with MAT patients. Mariya, who was receiving treatment in Kyiv, described a similar gap between her desires for herself and her personal control over her drug use:

> You know, there are some people who like drinking. They like the feeling. I don't. I never enjoyed the feeling of being drunk. I did other things. But the purpose of all of it is just to relax a bit, right? But, unfortunately, it wasn't that kind of relaxation. It alters your perception of reality, making everything fluffy around the edges. And you have these moments where you realize that you're tired of all of it, tired of using, but you go out looking for more just the

same. You hunt, you buy, you cook, you shoot it up. You're even doing it when you have no veins left, even after you've been sitting for two or three hours looking for a place where the needle will hit.

This frustration, this sense of wanting to stop but simply having no control over one's use, is also apparent in Timur's recollection of his path in and out of different hospitals and treatment programs. "The point is not to raise your dose," he said. "But to lower it . . . I want to quit, but [the narcotics] are holding on too tightly to my body." Timur claims that he has a desire, but the nature of "addiction" makes it impossible for him to regain the control he needs to make that desire a reality. A key difference, however, is that these patients insist that they possess the desire to quit in spite of their failure to do well on MAT. For them, MAT can intervene on their daily logistical troubles, but not on the root psychological or biological elements of their drug use. As their clinicians mark them as failures, blaming their difficulties on a deep-seated indifference, patients frame their entire lived experience with drug use as saturated with unmet desires. They insist that, in the face of all this, they are doing the best that they can.

The Neighbor's Boy

As Sergey and I traveled around Ukraine together, we typically stayed in privately owned apartments, which were leased out on a nightly basis. This is a common practice for travelers in Eastern Europe, far predating the advent of "gig economy" travel services in the United States. When we arrived in the city of Kherson in the summer of 2013, we called around until we found an available flat and met the owner in the courtyard of the building where we would stay. Our interaction was typical. She gave us a tour of the place, wrote down the Wi-Fi password, and showed us the how to properly shake the handle on the toilet to keep the water from overflowing. When she asked us what we were doing in town, Sergey told her outright that we were there to visit the HIV hospital and discuss MAT, a treatment for substance use disorder, with the clinicians there. Sergey was always quite straightforward with things like this, paying no mind to the perceived social indignity he invited into "pleasant conversation" each time he mentioned these stigmatized topics.

Our temporary landlord wasn't scandalized by the comment; she was enraged. She told us that there were bad people at that hospital. She told us that a neighbor's boy—a good boy—went in for some kind of care, and the doctors "hooked" him on drugs and destroyed his family. Based on her description, neither Sergey nor I were ever able to gain a clear understanding of this young man's situation: why he had sought help, what he was being treated for, whether or not he had been using drugs to begin with. These pertinent details notwithstanding, our landlord's great distress that this young man was now "on drugs" and "lost" to his family and the community, was deep and palpable. He was taken, caught, consumed by these powerful substances. For the landlord, it was a tragedy of epic proportions. Sergey tried to respond to some of her accusations regarding the hospital and its staff, but he quickly relented, seeing that he was only upsetting her further.

The idea that "addiction" traps the will by forcing people to lose control of themselves looms large in the Ukrainian popular imagination, ascribing meaning to a vast array of behaviors, urges, and states of consciousness. Our landlord in Kherson put these ideas into action. In her mind, her neighbor's son had been robbed of his free will by being given and then "hooked" on drugs. Likewise, many clinicians characterized patients who are struggling or are failing to progress into abstinence from illicit drug use as lacking the fundamental desire to do so. Timur and Lyuda's insistence to the contrary, though, reveals the holes in this theory. Their testimonies show that the dominant psychological approach to substance use disorder in these crucial programs captures only some of the lived experiences they are meant to influence. Just as the accounting and audit practices endorsed by international donor institutions are transmuted into locally meaningful and useful bookkeeping systems (see chapter 2), so international approaches to harm reduction and treatment for substance use disorder also become situated within local discourses as they move across national and cultural boundaries.

At the time of my research, MAT clinicians in Ukraine were adopting a clear and prescriptive interpretation of this medical terrain where "addiction," psychology, and personhood intersect. Opioid-dependent people are seen as problematic and dangerous because "addiction," as many clinicians claim, can only arise in someone who is indifferent or lacks desire. Desire, in this view, is what connects people to their primary social roles and relationships. As a population that has been perceived as living in constant contradiction to those roles and relationships, people who use drugs require a unified explanation for their apparent pathology if they are to be socially understood. And if desire is seen as the first thing that motivates people into relationships, then the postulate that "addicts" fall out of those relationships due to a lack of desire would, in this view, make a good deal of sense. "Addiction" is, therefore, viewed as a negative state, because this lack of integration is what makes "addicts" troublesome, and it is precisely this that treatment efforts aim to resolve.

Patients like Timur and Lyuda, however, levied their own claims as well. They were both quick to take ownership of their self-management strategies and to defend the validity of their efforts. They presented themselves not as indifferent but as actively engaged in their own strategies of self-care. In other words, the clinical paradigm of "addiction" that has taken hold among the professionals operating Ukraine's MAT programs must be understood as a discourse that exists in concert, and occasionally in conflict, with a variety of strategies that people who use drugs adopt to manage their bodies, their identities, and their lives. However, as the remainder of this book will argue, there are many more who reject the possibility of such reintegration, whose "addiction imaginary" considers people who use drugs to be social "others" who need to be contained, controlled, and even eliminated for the welfare of the state and the subjects it governs.

Chapter 4

STAR WARS AND THE STATE

In the summer of 2010, Ukraine's president, Viktor Yanukovych, brought a collection of illegal drugs to a cabinet meeting. He had affixed little vials of the stuff to a folding display board, which looked not terribly unlike a high school science project. He claimed to have purchased all of these drugs, ranging from synthetic marijuana to powder cocaine, through online retailers. He said he had brought them to this meeting to demonstrate how poorly the leaders of the state police were controlling drug trafficking into the country. After publicly excoriating various high-ranking officials in attendance, Yanukovych carried his contraband out onto the stone courtyard of the parliament building where he was met by an emergency fire brigade and a cadre of news reporters. As the cameras rolled and the fire fighters stood watch, he threw the vials into a metal chute on top of some dry kindling and proceeded, rather anticlimactically, to try to set the whole lot on fire.

I had lunch with my friend Ivan the day after all this appeared on local television. When he sat down across from me, he was visibly upset, smoking more frequently and urgently than usual. After working for several years as an English translator for the Alliance, Ivan was very familiar with patterns of drug use across Ukraine and the true public health consequences of those behaviors. "This thing Yanukovych did," he told me between long drags on a cigarette, "this is the sign of an imbecile. The people who are most at risk, and are the hardest hit by the [HIV] epidemic—this is not how they buy drugs. These people [high-risk people who use drugs], they do not even know what cocaine is."

Ivan's anger was directed, first, at the prevalence of misinformation about drug use in Ukraine. Such inaccurate beliefs, like those projected by Yanukovych's theatrics, can be particularly problematic for staff at the Alliance, because the very MAT and harm reduction programs they try to buoy up are founded upon the belief that substance use disorders are fundamentally biomedical conditions. This narrow, scientific view is directly opposed to cultural narratives that frame substance use as a sign of moral degradation and social peril (Singer and Page 2013; Valverde 1998). Second, Ivan was also frustrated with the use of drugs and, by extension, Ukrainians who use them as props in self-serving acts of political theater. He was especially offended that the president chose to air his grievances with the state police by invoking negative and inaccurate social images of people who use drugs. Rather than speaking to the realities of substance use, Yanukovych used *the idea* of people who use substances as harmful and dangerous for the purpose of publicly shaming his political subordinates.

Engaging with a shared "addiction imaginary" to express a larger social or political message is a relatively common strategy in Ukraine—as it is in many other parts of the world. Some contemporary examples are grandiose, such as the public characterization of opponents of the Orange Revolution in 2004 (Fournier 2012) and, later, of the Maidan revolution in 2014 (Carroll 2016a) as drug-addled idiots who were out on the streets because they were too high to know what they were doing (see chapter 5). Others are more subtle, such as the complaints made by nurses I met in TB hospitals that their most truant patients were all useless *narkomany* who would never present themselves to the clinic for care (see chapter 3). All these examples evoke an "addiction imaginary" (a culturally contingent stereotype that defines people who use drugs as deficient in individual will) in the service of a larger social or political message: the police force is obligated to protect its citizens and its borders; participants in the popular revolution are not simply bad people, they are also psychologically damaged (by drugs); *narkomany* are cavalier with their health, therefore someone who is cavalier with his health must be some kind of *narkoman*. Collectively, these discourses endorse a set of ideological values about how good citizens should act and how a strong, successful state should care for the enfranchised in the face of both internal and external dangers.

Two recent examples of political discourse in Ukraine engaged "addiction imaginaries" to levy such claims: one rooted in diplomacy, the other in parody. The first of these acts took place in a lengthy correspondence between the MoH and the Alliance. In March 2012, Ukraine's MoH passed a new law, Order 200, which established tight restrictions on access to MAT, stipulating that only people who had failed multiple attempts at "ordinary" or medication-free forms of therapy (like talk therapy) would be eligible to access this form of care. This new policy was a clear violation of international standards and threatened the country's grant agreement with the Global Fund. In response, the Alliance quickly began lobbying the MoH in writing, imploring them to nullify the new regulation. With both parties adopting the role of a national authority on health care and the body politic of Ukraine, they entered into a debate about the responsibilities of the state toward its citizens and whether (or how) people who use drugs should be included among them.

The second example comes from the Internet Party of Ukraine, a political party led by young adults from the city of Odessa. Many of this party's leaders have legally changed their names to those of *Star Wars* characters: Darth Vader, Chewbacca, and Yoda, among others. They dress in costume, prank government officials, and post viral videos of their antics online. Exploiting the current nadir of confidence in the Ukrainian government, the Internet Party's actions have resonated with many of Ukraine's youth and propelled them to minor pop-culture fame. Of interest to this analysis is that many of their posted videos touch on issues of drug use, the illegal drug market, and the moral imperative of the government to eradicate socially toxic *narkomany* from the enfranchised population. They have delivered mock legislation to the Cabinet of Ministers and carried out unsanctioned "raids" against alleged "drug dens" in their hometown. Part political theater, part genuine activism, these activists criticize the inaction of local and state governments by satirically performing the duties of the government themselves.

Insofar as both of these public conversations took place within the problem space of citizenship and sovereignty, they both illustrate how people who use drugs can be good to think with when articulating social values about the state and society. These public acts are concerned not simply with articulating the ideals of citizenship or the entitlements promised therein, but also with reifying the boundary between the enfranchised and the disenfranchised and describing how the state is morally obliged to interact with individuals in either group. In the discursive spaces created by these public performances, *narkomany* (as a distinct group) are evoked to mean many different things and are imbued with different social values. They are defined by various actors as citizens, as noncitizens, and as threats to public welfare at different times and in different places, and each view generates different understandings of citizenship and the role of the government.

Also important are the accidental congruencies that can occur between the medicalized subject-position of people who use drugs—specifically that upon which the logic of MAT as a remedy for substance-use disorder is founded—and the perceived social substrate of drug-using actors in Ukrainian popular imagination (the "addiction imaginary"). When social and medical discourses meet, the concept of *"narkoman"* or "addict" acts as a boundary object, an idea that varies in its meaning across contexts. The term can be legitimately used in both discourses but does not carry the same meaning across them. When the signifier is used, the meaning evoked in the mind of the audience will vary according to what discourse he or she has adopted. As a result of this plasticity in the "addiction imaginary," it is difficult for public-health advocates to refer to "people who use drugs as citizens with a right to health care" without local actors thinking about "people who use drugs as noncitizens who represent a social threat." As the accounts in this chapter illustrate, defending the first can reinforce the apparent validity of the second.

Drug Use as Exception

Many current anthropological theories of citizenship consider how neoliberal market forces shape the way that states govern and that citizenship rights are apportioned and received. Aihwa Ong has described these shifts as the disarticulation and subsequent rearticulation of "the elements that we think of as coming together to create citizenship—rights, entitlements, territoriality, a nation" (Ong 2006, 7). In places that have not necessarily followed the

Western trend of hyperindividualism, she argues, these rearrangements of citizenship and sovereignty are invoked in moments of exception, moments in which market logic and the interests of private capital require a new configuration of the social order to optimize the labor power of certain portions of the population. In Ukraine, the processes that Ong describes are certainly taking place across many sectors of society. The fact that foreign technology companies offer between UAH 15,000 and UAH 20,000 per month (USD 586–782 at the time of writing) to software developers, yet the average teacher working in higher education is provided a monthly salary of only UAH 3,000 (USD 117 at the time of writing) is a clear example of the inequitable distribution of rights and protections across the labor market. However, in Ukraine, where the legacy of Soviet rule lingers in the not-too-distant past, other ideals of statehood and citizenship continue to have purchase across many aspects of social and political life.

The relationship of the state to its citizens during the Soviet era has often been criticized as overly paternalistic, nurturing the development of "homo Sovieticus" (Zinoviev 1985), a citizen-subject who is passive and dependent to the point of self-harm, expecting all the comforts of life to be delivered by the state. In reality, Soviet paradigms of citizenship and sovereignty were much more nuanced than this. In the context of a centrally planned society, Soviet citizens participated in social structures that were intimately linked with (and mutually dependent upon) the physical and political infrastructure of the Union. Stephen Collier, for example, has noted that entire cities were designed during the Soviet period to impart just the right amount of order and flexibility to the residents' interconnected social roles (Collier 2011). Likewise, personal relationships grew and evolved not only to fulfill basic psychosocial needs but also to play key roles in the distribution of finances and material goods across the population (Dunn 2004; Ledeneva 2006; Parsons 2014; Patico 2008). These social ties allowed Soviet citizens not only to "get by" but sometimes even to thrive within an economy of deficit. To accurately characterize this configuration of society, it is not enough to say that citizens relied on the government for elements of their well-being. Rather, as citizens got on with their daily lives, the state was defined and justified by the specific obligations it had toward those citizens, and vice versa. Providing certain services for the welfare of the population was—and often still is—seen as the entire purpose of having an organized government in the first place. The question to be answered, then, is how some people's social status as *narkomany* affects their citizenship status and the rights to which they are entitled.

Interestingly, much foundational anthropological work at the intersection of health and citizenship has been based on ethnographic research carried out in Ukraine in the 1990s. Adriana Petryna introduced the term "biological citizenship" into the medical anthropological lexicon in her book, *Life Exposed*, a moving ethnography of Ukrainian victims of the Chernobyl disaster. Petryna defines biological citizenship as "a massive demand for but selective access to a form of social welfare based on medical, scientific, and legal criteria that both acknowledge biological injury and compensate for it" (Petryna 2002, 6). She illustrates this point through the experiences of some individuals who chose to expose themselves to radiation following the Chernobyl disaster in order to improve the likelihood that the effects of radiation would be clinically visible. Most of these individuals were already sick and suffering the consequences of radiation exposure, but not severely enough for the state to acknowledge them as injured and grant them access to the social welfare and support systems specifically designated for Chernobyl victims.

Even now, everyday life in Ukraine remains colored by the perceived obligation of the state to provide certain forms of care for its most deserving citizens—the very perception that inspired Petryna's work among Chernobyl victims in the 1990s. In the summer of 2010, for example, I lived on the outskirts of Kyiv with a local family who all (except for the youngest daughter, who was not yet born in 1986 when the Chernobyl accident occurred) were officially classified by the state as "sufferers" of the disaster. My hostess, a middle-aged homemaker named Tania, proudly showed me the special documents that affirmed their status as "sufferers" (Ukr: *poterpyly*). She spoke with gravity about the ills they had suffered and the readiness with which the Ukrainian state afforded the health care they subsequently needed. Her pride in these services provided by the Ukrainian government was equally matched by her feelings of indignation for the Soviet state, which she said had done nothing for them. More than once during my short stay with her family, Tania and her children, now grown and raising children of their own, received evaluations at the local polyclinic as part of their welfare benefits. Tania also made sure I noticed the small scars her eldest daughter bore on the soft skin above her collarbone. These were the last traces of a thyroidectomy to remove a gland that turned cancerous in her childhood as a result of radiation exposure. The surgical procedure was provided free of charge by the state.

In her analysis of post-Chernobyl welfare, Petryna observed, "The linking of biology with identity is not new. What is new is how connections between biology and identity are being made" (Petryna 2002, 14). That emergent connection was solidified through state policies enacted shortly after Ukraine's independence from the Soviet Union. In a form of legislative backlash against the perceived neglect of Soviet citizens, the independent government lowered the levels of radiation exposure required to qualify for special medical services to 20 percent of that required by Soviet authorities. The newly independent government also imposed a 12 percent income tax on both state and private businesses to fund the new services promised to citizens who were owed social and medical compensation (Petryna 2002, 23–24). With the number of official suffers reaching 3.5 million by 1996 (which, at that time, was approximately 7 percent of Ukraine's total population), the Ukrainian state categorically lacked the financial ability to fulfill the promises it had made, and frequently placed the unmet needs of Chernobyl victims at the forefront of their appeals for financial support from the World Bank and other international monetary institutions (Petryna 2002, 101). Yet, as Tania's seriousness in explaining her family's medical care reveals, the financial impracticalities of these state provisions for Chernobyl victims have had little bearing on the perceived appropriateness or moral necessity of this benefit system, even decades after the disaster.

Though the forms of biologically mediated citizenship that Petryna analyzed were distinctly Ukrainian phenomena, other anthropologists of global health and medicine have seen similar entanglements between biomedical conditions and citizens' rights elsewhere—especially in the context of international responses to HIV. Since its emergence in the early 1980s, HIV has generally been treated as an exceptional disease. It has always borne some association with social deviance (i.e., drug use, sexual promiscuity, homosexuality), moral threat, or the limits of scientific technology to mitigate biological danger (Sontag 1988). By the 1990s, HIV ceased being defined as an exclusively "gay disease," and its relevance to the mainstream population became more widely acknowledged. Following this shift, targeted financial and regulatory responses to HIV sprang to life, producing new funding streams for treatment research, enhanced medical education on HIV and related diseases, and new standards of care for those living with HIV (Wakeman, Green, and Rich 2014). In addition to boosting the discovery of effective new treatments, these developments also effectively reclassified HIV as an exceptional sociomedical problem experienced by "worthy" citizens, one deserving special treatment, one whose patients required extraordinary care. Anthropologist Adia Benton has argued that the very financial structures and interventions intended to respond to the global HIV epidemic "entrench and reinforce HIV's exceptional status" (Benton 2015, 9). The end result of the exceptional status given to HIV, and to people living with HIV, was the establishment of single-purpose or "stove-piped" (Garrett 2007) medical programs, which brought HIV care to impoverished nations in a manner disconnected from broader medical aid or development assistance.

This variety of biomedical exceptionalism easily becomes entangled with local notions of sovereignty—that discursive space where the greatest social and political control lies—because the determination of who or what constitutes an exception rests, by definition, in the hands of sovereign powers. Physician and anthropologist Vinh-Kim Nguyen has described this ability to distinguish different forms of citizenship along biological lines, specifically, as "therapeutic sovereignty": the ability to determine through social and biomedical means who does and does not qualify as a special exception: who does and does not deserve the rights and privileges of "therapeutic citizenship" (Nguyen 2010, 6). However, whereas biological citizenship, in Petryna's conception, is rooted in the recognition of the individual as a biological exception by a state power and fulfilled in that individual's claims against that state for services to redress the individual's exceptional need, Nguyen's concept of therapeutic citizenship acknowledges the emergence of an international structure of governance (like the Global Fund), which, when correctly appealed to, may step in to offer necessary services that the state has failed to provide. In Ukraine both of these governing structures—national and international, governmental and nongovernmental—are present and deeply complicit in the provision of MAT for people who use drugs and the social implications of access to this form of care.

As the examples in this chapter reveal, many perceptions of sovereignty and of people who use drugs as an exceptional class can exist simultaneously, because the concept of "drug user" functions as a boundary object—a flexible concept that inhabits multiple social worlds at the same time. In their seminal study of communication between scientists, Susan Leigh Star and

James Griesemer define boundary objects as, "Objects, which are both plastic enough to adapt to local needs and the constraints of several parties employing them, yet robust enough to maintain a common identity across sites. They are weakly structured in common use, but become strongly structured in individual site use" (1989, 393). "Addiction," generally speaking, is this kind of boundary object. For the sake of illustration, consider the fact that several contradictory definitions of "addiction" can be identified across American society. It is simultaneously understood to be a personal weakness (Valverde 1998), a chronic relapsing brain disease (National Institute on Drug Abuse 2016), and a collection of social, psychological, and biological symptoms grouped together under a single diagnostic heading (American Psychiatric Association 2013). Any of these views may be invoked at one time or another depending on social or political necessity at the moment of utterance. Boundary objects are the very things that permit the biomedical frames of global health programs to "graft" onto preexisting social discourses in the local places where they operate. Thus, as agents of global health programs invoke Western, biomedical values to discuss at-risk populations, Ukrainian government representatives and public personalities invoke a different set of local values to define this group of people.

It is true that people who use drugs are not the only group in Ukraine marginalized by their behavior or lifestyles. Homosexual men continue to experience significant social and professional discrimination (Chybisov 2016). LGBTQ communities have also been subject to violent attacks, both opportunistically on the street and during organized LGBTQ pride parades in Kyiv in 2015 and 2016, the latter of which I took part in. Though significant progress remains to be made toward the full inclusion of LGBTQ people into Ukrainian society, I draw a distinction between the social marginalization of LGBTQ people and people who use drugs along the following lines: first, public perceptions of sexual minorities in Eastern Europe have been slowly improving since the mid-1990s (Gessen 2017). Human Rights Watch has noted that violence against LGBTQ events has declined in recent years (Human Rights Watch 2017a), and recently remarked that "the government [of Ukraine] has introduced several progressive policies supporting lesbian, gay, bisexual, and transgender (LGBT) people" despite continued anti-LGBTQ sentiments across government bodies (Human Rights Watch 2017b). In the 2010s, however, the same organization denounced what they described as Viktor Yanukovych's "heavy-handed tactics . . . targeting people who use drugs," alleging the following abuses: "Police have raided drug treatment clinics; interrogated, fingerprinted, and photographed patients; confiscated medical records and medications; and detained medical personnel in cities nationwide. Many raids appear to have been conducted without probable cause and in violation of Ukraine's rules for police operations" (Human Rights Watch 2011). Further, physicians in Ukraine have never been subject to arrest for serving homosexual patients, unlike physicians working in MAT clinics (see chapter 2).

Further, as I argued in chapter 3, "addiction imaginaries" congeal around perceived violations of dominant theories of the will among people who use drugs. Put another way, "addiction imaginaries" provide explanations for why people who use drugs appear to some to act with such little self-control and why they appear to suffer from a deficiency of individual will. LGBTQ people in Ukraine do not stand accused of suffering from the same deficiency. Many perceive them as "deviant," but in this case they are perceived as willful practitioners of their lifestyles, not as individuals devoid of personal agency. I thus argue that the "addiction imaginary" is robust enough to be deployed by numerous social actors in a variety of settings to make claims about sovereignty, citizenship, and the role of the state. This image can be used understandably and appropriately by all the actors in these dialogues but, when they engage with the term, none of them mean exactly the same thing. In this way, the Alliance's reference to people who use drugs as an exceptional class—even if they mean to indicate a class of individuals with inalienable rights—can lend credence to local ideas that people who use drugs are an exceptional class of a different, less worthy kind.

Order 200

Though MAT programs in Ukraine have historically been funded through grants from the Global Fund, the rules and regulations governing the provision of MAT are set by the Ukrainian government. Under the jurisdiction of the MoH, these protocols are regulated through a piece of legislation cataloged as MoH Order No. 200. This law was first approved on March 27, 2012, and ratified later that summer. It has since undergone several revisions, the most recent of which was ratified on December 17, 2015. This order outlines the national standards for MAT care, specifying eligibility criteria for patients, outlining physicians' scope of practice within the context of MAT care, and detailing the formal reporting procedures required of MAT clinics. It was drafted and enacted as part of the MoH's fulfillment of its 2009–13 National HIV Control Strategy (Ministry of Health of Ukraine 2015), making it a key regulatory component of the state's public health infrastructure.

When first drafted in 2012, Order 200 imposed strict requirements on the administration of MAT programs. It mandated various reporting mechanisms for physicians that many found to be unreasonable, redundant, or unclear. The MoH also stipulated that the decision to make a diagnosis of opioid use disorder (as well as the subsequent decision to initiate MAT for any given patient) could only be made by a commission of at least three licensed narcologists—a requirement impossible to fulfill in most of Ukraine, where a single narcologist is typically present to serve the population of a large rural area (see chapter 2). For patients, Order 200 required, among other things, a history of at least three years of illicit drug use before initiating treatment as well as official documentation of two failed attempts at treatment without medication assistance (Ukr: *likuvannia bez zastosuvannia narkotychnykh zasobiv*) in a regional narcology clinic within the past year (Ministry of Health of Ukraine 2015). The order did not specify what constituted acceptable forms of treatment, acceptable forms of documentation, or sufficient evidence that a treatment attempt had "failed." In this way, Order 200 effectively prevented the use of MAT as a first-line treatment for opioid use disorder and forced patients and physicians to proactively demonstrate that each instance of treatment was genuinely "necessary," per the MoH's definition.

I first learned of Order 200 in the fall of 2012, about three months after it had gone into effect. I was traveling with Sergey in the southern city of Kherson, the same place where we infuriated our landlord by mentioning our intentions to visit a local MAT program (see chapter 3). While stopping by a tiny polyclinic on the outskirts of town, we met a physician who told us of a narcologist colleague in the city of Kharkiv who had devised a special plan for dealing with the order. The doctor and his staff would allegedly enroll patients in an accelerated "recovery program" that lasted about two weeks. This recovery program was designed to fail. By helping patients complete and fail two such treatment programs in rapid succession, the clinic could legally produce the documents necessary for their opioid-dependent patients to qualify for MAT in about a month's time. Though logistically awkward, this pathway to MAT effectively reduced delays in care for their patients' down to a little more than thirty days. By most standards, this is an unacceptably long time to postpone the initiation of treatment for someone who needs and wants MAT. In the context of the new Order 200, however, this process seemed virtually streamlined. Though I had no way to independently confirm the truth behind this story, I was struck by how plausible the physician in Kherson found it to be. In the face of ridiculous barriers to care, ridiculous work-arounds seemed a reasonable thing to implement.

Distaste for the restrictions imposed by Order 200 was not limited to physicians seeking to connect their patients with treatment. The Alliance also began formally protesting the content of the original order within weeks of its passing. They continued their lobbying campaign for the better part of a year, until, under significant pressure from both local and international agencies, the MoH finally amended its regulation. Until that time, representatives from the Alliance not only attended regular stakeholder meetings with the MoH where they advocated their position, they also took part in lengthy correspondence with various government entities to lobby for the order's revision. What became clear over the course of that correspondence was that the fundamental disagreement between the MoH and the Alliance was not over whether Order 200 allowed MAT programs to serve their purposes properly, but over what that purpose actually was. They further disagreed about what sort of citizen-subject position people who use drugs could occupy, how the government should treat people in that subject position, and how MAT fulfilled that obligation.

In a letter dated May 16, 2012, the Alliance delivered its first words of concern to Raisa Bogatyrova, who was then serving as both minister of health and vice prime minister of Ukraine.[1] Their initial objections were practical: the new requirements for eligibility would limit Ukrainians' access to treatment, thus preventing the country from reaching its own goal of scaling up MAT to meet the goals of its own HIV control strategy:

> It is our responsibility to inform you that your signing of the revised technical components of MoH Order 200 has rendered impossible the implementation of the 2009–2013 National Program for HIV Prevention and Treatment and the Care and Support of Those Living with HIV and AIDS, which became law on November 19, 2009 (No. 1026-IV), which stipulated that 20,000

people who inject drugs would receive MAT by the end of 2013. Moreover, the number of patients already receiving MAT is at risk of declining under the current revisions to the order.[2]

Reaching 20,000 patients would have required a 150 percent increase in the volume of treatment coverage at that time (Bojko, Dvoriak, and Altice 2013). Furthermore, the Alliance argued, burdensome and sometimes contradictory reporting requirements put physicians at risk for criminal prosecution. This threat felt particularly immediate following the 2010 arrests of two MAT physicians, Yaroslav Olendr in Ternopil' and Ilya Podolyan in Odessa, who were charged with drug trafficking for activities they carried out in the normal course of providing patient care (see chapter 2).

In addition to voicing concern over these matters, the Alliance emphasized to the vice prime minister that the contents of Order 200 might affect Ukraine's international reputation. First and foremost, they argued, the order represented a step backward in Ukraine's attempts to conform to international standards of health care, thereby potentially jeopardizing Ukraine's relationship with the Global Fund. Furthermore, they wrote, by ostensibly limiting Ukrainians' constitutionally protected right to health care, the ratification of Order 200 "may tarnish Ukraine's international image as a democratic state, which upholds human rights and fulfills its international obligations." To substantiate these claims, the Alliance attached to their letter a seventeen-page document detailing the text of the order, their recommended changes to the text, and a lengthy rationale for every proposed edit. In this enclosed document, Alliance staff appealed multiple times to the rights of all Ukrainian citizens to health care, as stipulated in the constitution of Ukraine, and the government's obligation to uphold it.

Though it had already made its position on the matter clear through the ratification of Order 200, the MoH nevertheless carried out its due diligence and responded to the Alliance in writing. In a letter dated May 29, 2012, the head of the MoH's State Service on HIV/AIDS and Other Socially Dangerous Diseases, Tetyana Alexandrina, agreed to remove the requirement that the two failed treatment attempts be carried out in state narcological institutions, but retained these prior failures as mandatory for MAT eligibility. She also agreed to reinstate priority enrollment for MAT seekers who had also been diagnosed with HIV, TB, hepatitis B, hepatitis C, sepsis, or cancer.[3] Aside from this, however, the MoH and other representative government bodies repeatedly insisted through their correspondence with the Alliance that Order 200 was, in fact, congruent with Ukraine's National Drug Control Strategy, Ukraine's National HIV Control Strategy, and the articles of the European Convention on Human Rights, and therefore required no redaction. Such a claim was made by the deputy minister of justice of Ukraine, Dmytro Vorona, in a letter to the Alliance dated June 18, 2012:

> The Ministry of Justice . . . confirms that the order taken by the MoH is in accordance with item 8, part 1, article 4 of the Ukrainian law "On countering the spread of diseases caused by the human immunodeficiency virus (HIV) and the legal and social protection for people living with HIV," item 2, section II of the appendix of the National Program for HIV Prevention and Treatment and the Care and Support of Those Living with HIV and AIDS, which became law on November 19, 2009 (No. 1026-IV), in agreement with the State Service for Drug Control.[4]

Another claim came from the first deputy minister of justice, Inna Emelyanova, in a letter dated July 17, 2012 to a physician who was providing MAT and had written in solidarity with the Alliance's protests:

> The order in question was standardized to item 8, part 1, article 4 of the Ukrainian law "On countering the spread of diseases caused by the human immunodeficiency virus (HIV) and the legal and social protection for people living with HIV," item 2, section II of the appendix of the National Program for HIV Prevention and Treatment and the Care and Support of Those Living with HIV and AIDS, which became law on November 19, 2009 (No. 1026-IV), in agreement with the State Service for Drug Control.[5]

And yet another claim like this from Emelyanova came in a letter to the Alliance dated November 5, 2012:

> The order in question was standardized to item 8, part 1, article 4 of the Ukrainian law "On countering the spread of diseases caused by the human immunodeficiency virus (HIV) and the legal and social protection for people living with HIV," item 2, section II of the appendix of the National Program for HIV Prevention and Treatment and the Care and Support of Those Living with HIV and AIDS, which became law on November 19, 2009 (No. 1026-IV), in agreement with the State Service for Drug Control.[6]

Government representatives toed this line so faithfully, in fact, that the text declaring Order 200's continuity with other legislation appears to be copied verbatim in these and each subsequent occurrence.

Seeing their appeals for citizens' right to health care regardless of whether they use drugs so resoundingly ignored, the Alliance quickly switched gears and began focusing instead on the importance of MAT for HIV control in the general population. In response to Tetyana Alexandrina's letter dated May 29, 2012, the Alliance sent her another written document on June 21.[7] In this letter, the Alliance took pains to emphasize that the stabilization of substance use disorder with MAT was necessary for successful HIV/AIDS treatment, and that active substance use should never serve as a barrier to care among those living with HIV. They wrote, "The treatment of opioid use disorder is an important part of care for HIV-positive individuals who inject drugs. HIV infection and opioid dependency are not separate, but exacerbate one another."[8] In their estimation, the requirement that individuals with substance use disorder undergo (and subsequently fail) two non-medication-assisted attempts at recovery before beginning MAT directly and negatively impacted HIV care by delaying the achievement of that stability and adding stress to the life of an HIV-positive person at the most critical time: when they are first initiated into HIV treatment. As a consequence, these patients would remain infectious for longer than necessary, increasing the risk that HIV would be transmitted and spread further to the general population.

The Alliance also lobbied the president of Ukraine, Viktor Yanukovych, directly about these HIV-related concerns. In a letter dated November 29, 2012, the Alliance asked him to fully fund treatment for HIV, TB, and hepatitis in Ukraine, and to prioritize the scale-up of MAT across the country. They wrote:

On November 13, 2012, you publicly stated that the government was responsible for fully financing programs to treat HIV/AIDS, tuberculosis [TB], and hepatitis and programs to prevent the spread of infectious disease. Today, on the eve of World AIDS Day, and as the draft for next year's state budget is being finalized, we once again call on you as head of state to take all possible legal measures to fully allocate the funds needed (923million UAH) to support the National Plan for HIV/AIDS in 2013. Hundreds of thousands of ill people and representatives of groups responsible for HIV as well as many engaged [Ukr: *nebaiduzhikh*] organizations are hoping to receive information from you about these expenditures in the 2013 budget, which the government will be finalizing next month for ratification by the Parliament of Ukraine.[9]

In their closing lines, the Alliance appealed to the president to personally ensure the provision of adequate health care for all Ukrainian citizens: "Saving the lives and the health of citizens should be a top priority for the government," they wrote. People living with HIV, the letter implies, are members of that citizenry, which the government is obligated to serve, especially if Ukraine is to live up to its desired reputation as a successful, functioning, democratic state.

Even though they spoke of MAT as a basic component of the health care the government is constitutionally obligated to provide, the way the Alliance defined that constitutionally enfranchised citizenry slowly transformed over the course of the correspondence. In their initial letters to Raisa Bogatyrova and in their first document of proposed changes sent to Tetyana Alexandrina,[10] the Alliance clearly outlines the benefits of MAT *for people who use drugs.* "It is important to remember that the stabilization of opioid use disorder in people who inject drugs with the help of MAT is a key component of the successful treatment of HIV/AIDS, including HAART [highly active antiretroviral therapy]. Active drug use should not interfere with HIV treatment."[11] Yet, in their subsequent letter to Alexandrina, they turn away from the need of these individuals for access to MAT and toward the general population's need for good HIV control. This turn began with the following claim: "Treatment for opioid use disorder is a key component of care for HIV-infected people who use drugs. HIV-infection and opioid dependence are not separate; they augment one another." From this point on, the Alliance's rhetorical strategy ceases to give voice to people who use drugs and instead aims to buoy government concern over a generalized HIV epidemic.

It was certainly reasonable for the Alliance to advocate for better HIV care in general. Such demands needed to be made, and the connections that they drew between quality MAT provision and quality HIV control are very real. However, just as not all people who use drugs are living with HIV, not all people living with HIV are also experiencing opioid use disorder and would benefit from MAT. There is overlap between these populations, but their membership, public image, and relationship to the rest of society are not the same. In other words, the nature of these groups' biomedical exceptionalism

is different, and the rights that the Ukrainian government was willing to acknowledge for each were different as well. Ultimately, what occurred in the
evolution of the Alliance's rhetorical tactics, as they began to make appeals
on behalf of a more "worthy" group, was a gradual conformity to the idea
that people who use drugs are unworthy of government concern, that they
are anti-citizens who do not (or do not deserve to) enjoy the same protections
and privileges as everyone else.

At this point, I want to state unequivocally that I am not criticizing the
Alliance for adapting its rhetorical strategies in this way. This was a very delicate situation with serious consequences; representatives of this organization were forced to make difficult choices while fighting difficult battles.
These strategic choices ultimately helped them to win this fight a year later
when the most problematic provisions were removed from Order 200. That
success is hugely commendable. What I want to draw attention to, however,
is that the strategy the Alliance fell back onto tacitly reproduced the marginalization of people who use drugs by distinguishing them from "ordinary"
Ukrainians as a potentially dangerous Other. The Alliance accomplished this
by appealing to the notion that the ordinary, enfranchised citizens of Ukraine
would benefit from better HIV control systems—including MAT—thereby
subordinating any discussion of what people who use drugs, as individuals
or as a population, needed for their own, individual well-being.

Though this strategy also created the potential to reinforce HIV-related
stigma, the Alliance had ample reason to find this outcome unlikely. In the
preceding years, HIV testing for key populations, including commercial sex
workers and gay men, had increased significantly; government funding for
HIV treatment had increased; and the MoH had passed new legislation to
improve the treatment of HIV/TB coinfection and strengthen the entire con-
tinuum of HIV care (WHO Regional Office for Europe 2013). The battle
for Ukrainian citizens' access to HIV care was already being won. It was
when the Alliance tried to frame people who use drugs as a part of the citizenry deserving of similar access to health care services that the MoH pushed
back. The key point here is this: in its efforts to advocate for the human rights
of Ukrainians who use drugs, representatives from the Alliance correctly understood that a tacit acknowledgment of the social value of "ordinary citizens" over "people who use drugs" was the only discernible path to success
in this particular battle.

These uneven or "variegated" citizenship categories (Ong 2006) can also be seen in the MoH's own statements about the logic behind the original provisions of Order 200. Rather than prioritizing the improved quality of life that MAT can offer to people struggling with opioid use disorder, government representatives tended to highlight the benefits MAT offered to the rest of society, benefits achieved by corralling people who use drugs inside therapeutic institutions and away from others. For example, in her May 29 letter to the Alliance, Tatiana Alexandrina refused to remove the following grounds for the termination of MAT from the revised Order 200, as the Alliance had requested: (1) "the attempt to remove MAT medications from clinic premises"; (2) "the initiation of a sentence from the courts or administrative procedure"; and (3) "the confirmation by urine test of the presence of drugs in the patient's bodily system."[12] She justified the inclusion of these criteria by articulating, in her words, the goals of MAT:

1. To decrease the use of illegal opioids by preventing the emergence of opioid withdrawal syndrome.
2. To stabilize and improve of the psychosomatic state of the opioid-dependent patient.
3. To decrease criminal activities related to injection drug use.
4. To decrease risk behaviors associated with the spread of HIV infection, hepatitis B and C, and other [blood diseases] among people who inject drugs.
5. To attract people who inject drugs into contact with social services and to create conditions for the social rehabilitation and reintegration of these patients into society.
6. To create conditions for the effective treatment of AIDS, TB, and accompanying illnesses of HIV (sepsis, purulent infections, hepatitis B and C, trophic ulcers, phlebitis).
7. To create conditions for quality medical services for pregnant women who use drugs.[13]

It is worth noting that the vast majority of these practical justifications for MAT actually benefit someone other than the MAT patient—with the exception, perhaps, of item numbers 2 and 6. Decreasing crime benefits society at large. Decreasing the risk of new HIV and hepatitis infections also benefits citizens who have not yet come into contact with the disease. Even care for pregnant women can, especially in a pronatalist political environment, be motivated largely by concern for the welfare of the child. One genuine benefit unique to the MAT patient acknowledged herein is the general improvement of the patient's mental and physical state—a relatively minor accomplishment considering the true range of benefits that MAT can provide to someone who needs it.

This belief that MAT is justified by the benefit it offers to those who are not patients appears throughout many of the government's letters to the Alliance. The deputy minister of health, Oleksandr Tolstanov, doubled down on this claim in his letter dated September 24, 2012. In defense of the MoH's work in drafting Order 200, he observed: "The State Service on HIV/AIDS and Other Socially Dangerous Diseases of Ukraine has taken great care in the preparation and approval of the Order, and, in addition to the interests of MAT patients, has also taken into account *the rights of Ukrainian citizens who do not inject drugs*"[14] (emphasis added). Furthermore, any suggestion on Tetyana Alexandrina's part that MAT is, indeed, offered for the benefit of Ukrainians with opioid use disorder is undermined by her insistence that legal proceedings and relapse into opioid use be grounds for the termination of care. Relapse and incarceration indicate that patients need a higher, not lower, level of care. The withdrawal of care in these circumstances can only be interpreted as punitive, not therapeutic. The population to be managed by MAT programs and the population against whose well-being the costs and benefits of MAT would be weighed were not one and the same (Mason 2016). According to MoH officials, people who use drugs were to be managed, but managed in a way that best served Ukraine's deserving, non-drug-using citizens.

Ultimately, both the Alliance and various entities in the Ukrainian government presented MAT as a key point of interaction between the state and certain segments of its population—a place where the government could act in fulfillment of its obligations toward its citizens in one way or another. However, the Alliance and the MoH imagined the limits of that citizenry and the subsequent citizen-subject positions into which people who use drugs were slated quite differently. Consequently, the obligations each organization perceived the state to hold toward those subjects, so defined, varied as well. Though the Alliance did not ultimately endorse the definition of people who use drugs as less worthy, neither were they able to push back against this idea while still protecting their fragile access to MAT. They only found success in their lobbying efforts through their tacit acceptance of a discourse that codes people who use drugs as noncitizens against which the rest of the body politic should be protected.

The Rise of the Dark Side

Around the time that politicians and public health advocates were occupied with the conflict over Order 200, a small group of political activists from the city of Odessa were gaining local celebrity. They called themselves the Internet Party of Ukraine. They first came together as a group in 2007, drafted their social platform in 2009 (Internet Party of Ukraine 2009a) and then formally registered as an official political party in Ukraine in 2010. At that time, the political landscape in Ukraine was crowded; they became Ukraine's 174th officially registered party (Interfax-Ukraine 2010). Their political platform lent support to high-tech reforms such as electronic voting, digital signature systems, full computer access for state schools and institutions, electronic management and funds transfer for social welfare and pension payments, electronic medical records, and free Wi-Fi for all (Internet Party of Ukraine 2009b).

The Internet Party of Ukraine is better described as a troupe of protest artists than as a functioning political party; registering with the Ministry of Justice and making humorous yet unsuccessful bids for local office simply adds a layer of authenticity to their satire. Party members often dress up as well-known characters from George Lucas's classic *Star Wars* saga and attempt to conduct business with local and state authorities as these personae. The most well-known of these performer-activists—and the official "leader" of the Internet Party—is an individual who cosplays as the nefarious villain Darth Vader. This Darth Vader impersonator consistently (and convincingly) presents his character as a true defender of Ukrainian values and an unquestionable authority on the health of the nation. He has hyperbolically performed this Darth Vader's Ukrainianness in popular online videos, such as one that depicts him playing the bandura (a classic Ukrainian stringed instrument) while sitting with his horse under a blossoming cherry tree—a highly recognizable trope associated with Ukrainian Cossack warriors.[15] In a different but related video, Darth Vader removes his black helmet to

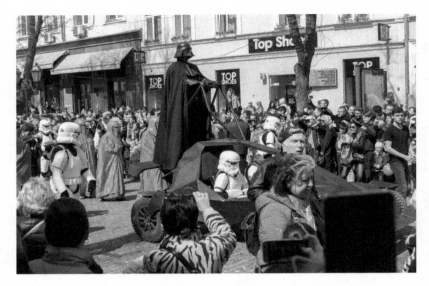

Darth Vader and other members of the Internet Party of Ukraine take part in the 2017 annual Humor Festival, a celebration of humor and satire, in Odessa, Ukraine. Photo by Cebanu Ghenadie. Source: https://www.flickr.com/photos/g23/33102448243/in /album-72157680589054030/.

reveal a distinctly Cossack hairstyle underneath.[16] The political messages conveyed in these videos are typically critiques of the Ukrainian government. For example, the video of Darth Vader playing the bandura under the cherry tree poked fun at the Ukrainian parliament's reputation for corruption with a voice-over track that says, "Don't let them eat our salo" (Ukr: *Ne damo z'yisty nashoho sala*). Salo is cured pork fat—a cherished national dish and a potent symbol of the national livelihood allegedly being stripped away from Ukrainians by their corrupt government officials.

Throughout its history, the Internet Party of Ukraine has engaged in numerous public displays that draw attention to one particular social issue and the state's failure to address it: drug use and drug trafficking in Ukraine. For example, on June 3, 2013, the party uploaded a video to its YouTube channel showing Darth Vader marching up Kyiv's Hrushevsky Street, flanked by more than a dozen storm troopers, toward the building of the Cabinet of Ministers of Ukraine to seek an audience with Prime Minister Mykola Azarov.[17] In the video, Darth Vader and his entourage are quickly stopped by guards in the driveway of the building. He introduces himself with theatrical gravitas to each new security officer he encounters: "I am Darth Vader, right hand of the Emperor Palpatine." Surrounded by a growing cluster of confused security officers, Vader forcefully demands to speak with Azarov on "topics related to the future of millions of Ukrainians." The guards watching over this government building are diligent in refusing him passage, resulting in several minutes of nonsensical back-and-forth between them. After a few moments, one of the officers on hand asks Darth Vader and his men to please step aside and out of the driveway and onto the sidewalk. Vader bites back: "You can't just tell Darth Vader where to go! How do you not get this? I am a Sith Lord. And who do you think you are?" The officer sighs in defeat, and bystanders can be heard laughing at the absurdity they are witnessing on the street.

The scene ends with a dour and harassed-looking bureaucrat emerging from the Cabinet of Ministers building to receive Darth Vader's written statement. After again offering his verbose introduction, Darth Vader expounds to this new representative about the troubles that he and his "constituents" are experiencing in Odessa:

> You have heard of the problems in Ukraine. In particular, in Odessa, people are engaging in the legal sale of narcotics. It goes on day and night all along Glushko Street. And I would like to see not only these elements, which operate openly in Odessa, removed, but to see such elements removed across all of Ukraine. Because with you all, here in Kyiv, I have not seen these kinds of stalls where they are selling these mixtures that are not included on the list of prohibited narcotic compounds, yet this situation does damage to the health of every Ukrainian.

Darth Vader then hands over his written statement to the suited man in front of him. Rather than accepting the document, the bureaucrat ignores Darth Vader's outstretched hand and coolly asks him why he has not simply taken up this issue with the police. Darth Vader replies that the police in Odessa are lining their own pockets with this drug trade. "Those who work as drug barons keep our state services in their pockets to protect their own interests," he says. "Everyone knows this."

About a week later, this group engaged in another disruptive act, this time in their hometown of Odessa. On this second occasion, they stormed a business on Pushkinska Street, which they claimed was selling narcotic products. A local news clip shows Darth Vader and several uniformed storm troopers throwing smoke bombs into the store, effectively flushing out the staff who were there.[18] In another scene, storm troopers hurl stones into the store and holler "For the Empire! A drug-free Ukraine!" (Rus: *Za emperii! Ukraina bez narkotikov!*). Some were filmed spray-painting stencils of Darth Vader's helmeted visage on the exterior of the building. A news anchor from Podrobnosti.ua, which reported the event, quoted a member of the raiding party as saying, "The police know all about [the drug sales], but they do nothing about it."

The Internet Party raided yet another location—an alleged "drug den" housing an illegal narcotics trade—in November of the same year. Darth Vader again made an appearance, as did Chewbacca and a handful of storm troopers. This time, however, the Internet Party gang was also accompanied by several dozen ominously dressed young men, most of them hiding their faces behind balaclavas or surgical masks. In a video posted by the Odessa-based news group Civil Alliance,[19] Darth Vader is shown marching with a megaphone, leading the group of rough-and-tumble-looking young men down the street as they chant in call-and-response style, "Ukraine! Without Drugs! Ukraine! Without Drugs!" (Rus: *Ukraina! Bez Narkoty!*). The actual attack was much more violent than the one they carried out in June. Their target was not a storefront, but a noncommercial rental unit with a street-facing entrance that was locked up tightly. The group began banging with sticks on the metal railings and walls around the entryway as someone used an angle grinder to saw through deadbolts and open the door. Responding to the ruckus, several police officers soon arrived to the location of the raid, and a substantial crowd of onlookers gathered around to watch the scene unfold.

It quickly became clear that the bystanders—ever growing in numbers—were delighted by what was happening. They cheered the raiding party on and yelled angrily at the dozen or so police officers who were trying in vain to keep the scene under control. In the video posted by Civil Alliance, a reporter moves through the crowd asking pedestrians to explain what they have seen there. "Why are the police showing up? What are they doing here?" she asks a woman on the sidewalk with her young child in tow. "The police are doing nothing here!" the woman replies. "They are all 'addicts' [*narkomany*] in that place." "And the police *protect* the *narkomany*!" a second woman shouts back. This response is echoed by many other members of the crowd, all of whom condemn the involvement of police forces in the local drug trade. Indeed, the most common refrain heard from angry residents was: "The police do nothing about *narkomany*. They do absolutely nothing at all."

Public reception of this satire, which frames the vicious and authoritarian leader of the fictional Galactic Empire as a morally righteous defender of the Ukrainian people, has been so positive because it cleverly taps into feelings of state abandonment harbored by many residents of Ukraine. On its face, the joke being played out here is that the Ukrainian government is so bad that even Darth Vader seems wonderful by comparison. As well, the level of absurdity that Internet Party members bring to their public stunts, including their commitment to their character roles when they go out in public, mirrors the absurdity that many Ukrainians see in their own parliament, which has been host to several physical brawls in recent years, including an infamous egg-throwing incident, which forced the speaker of the Parliament at the time, Volodymyr Lytvyn, to carry out his duties at the podium while guarded by two security officers carrying large umbrellas (Harding 2010).

On a deeper level, the Internet Party of Ukraine stages performances that diagnose specific ideological pathologies in the Ukrainian government. In their view, the role of the state is to protect its citizens from dangerous elements, and individuals who use drugs are viewed as the personification of those evils. Clearly, even as the Global Fund funnels millions of dollars into Ukraine to fund MAT for substance use disorder, and even as the Alliance debates the MoH over the human rights of people who use drugs, the diffusion of biomedical understandings of substance use into Ukrainian society remains demonstrably thin. Much of the population remains content to view people who use drugs as categorically intolerable, as dangerous creatures. It is this underlying belief that motivates the Internet Party's theatrical and sometimes aggressive actions against those they allege to be engaged in drug use. Their philosophy presumes an ideal relationship between the state and its citizens and draws on a significant "addiction imaginary" to accuse state authorities of failing to uphold their end of the bargain.

Power Putinesque

The exclusionary tactics adopted by the MoH and the Internet Party of Ukraine are but a repetition of similar activities that took place on the larger geopolitical landscape in the preceding decades. For example, toward the end of 1999, the year Vladimir Putin was elected to the Russian presidency, urban centers across Russia experienced a series of massive explosions in residential complexes—some of them deadly. Though there was little corroborating evidence, journalist Masha Gessen reports that everyone at the time "knew" that these acts had been carried out by Chechens, a Muslim minority living in a southern region of Russia near the Republic of Georgia. In fact, the preponderance of hard evidence then and now indicates that the explosions were part of a false-flag attack carried out by the Russian Security Service. Putin succeeded in harnessing Russian citizens' shared panic about the threat of outside attackers from Chechnya to consolidate power and renew questions regarding the difference between Russian and Soviet nationalism, or whether there was a difference at all (Gessen 2017). This discourse became a major theme of Putin's presidency. In his 2005 address to the Federal Assembly of the Russian Federation, he declared the collapse of the Soviet Union to be "the greatest geopolitical disaster of the [twentieth] century" (Putin 2005), and, upon returning to the presidential office in 2012, declared the reintegration of post-Soviet space to be one of his primary tasks (Plokhy 2017).

Putin made these priorities manifest beyond Russia's borders by involving the Russian military in numerous territorial conflicts in the Eastern European and Central Asian region. Residents of South Ossetia, a region in the Republic of Georgia, as well as residents of Transnistria in the Republic of Moldova, were fighting to secede and join Russia. Under the guise of providing protection to Russian-language speakers in these areas—people whom the Kremlin said it was duty-bound to protect—Russia sent military forces to support the separatist movements in each state, which has left its army mired in the business of propping up these de facto states still today (Gessen 2017). Anthropologists Elizabeth Dunn and Michael Bobick, who have conducted ethnographic research in South Ossetia and Transnistria, respectively, have argued that these military engagements were inspired less by a sense of loyalty for the people of the "Russian world" (Rus: *russkii mir*) who live beyond Russia's borders than out of concern for the growing affiliations between countries like Georgia, Moldova, Ukraine, and the European Union (EU). An association agreement between the EU and any of these countries would bring NATO, which many Russians still blame for the bombing of their Orthodox ally Serbia over the actions of the Yugoslav army in the predominantly Muslim region of Kosovo in 1999, uncomfortably close to Russian borders. These breakaway regions, then, served as "perches from which to threaten the states that once governed them" (Dunn and Bobick 2014, 406).

Until 2014, Russia succeeded in controlling its interests in Ukraine through different means. Rather than foment a separatist crisis, Russia was able to leverage its significant financial upper hand to influence Ukrainian politics. In the 1990s, metallurgic industries in the southeast of Ukraine made this region the country's most profitable economic sector and drove the creation of wealth among industry leaders in that area (including oligarchs such as Rinat Akhmetov, Viktor Pinchuk, and Igor Kolomoyski). Though natural gas was a major export for the Ukrainian SSR, Ukraine's gas fields had been all but depleted by the 1990s, leaving the country and its one profitable industry reliant on Russian gas imports (Plokhy 2017). By 1994, Ukraine was already seeking loans in the amount of USD 1.5 billion from the International Monetary Fund to pay its gas debts to Russia (Reid 1997). This power imbalance helped Russia bring Viktor Yanukovych, a politician from the southeastern Donbas region of Ukraine and an exceedingly manipulable man, to the Ukrainian presidency in 2010. Yanukovych's campaign succeeded by mobilizing Ukraine's eastern regions, where metallurgy and mining still dominate the economy, where reliance on Russian gas promoted a desire for good relations between the two countries, and where Yanukovych argued that the Russian language and the historical legacy of the Great Patriotic War (the name used in the Soviet Union for World War II) were under threat from European-influenced politicians in Kyiv (Plokhy 2017).

With a president so closely tied and so deeply indebted to Russia, the Kremlin was able to pull Ukraine farther away from any potential political or economic affiliations with the EU in subsequent years. That influence appears to be a significant factor in the 2012 amendments to MoH Order 200, which premised its new limitations on access to MAT for people who use drugs on its responsibility to "[take] into account the rights of Ukrainian citizens who do not inject drugs."[20] This position brought Order 200 into closer alignment with Russian domestic policy on illicit substance use, which affords little in the way of harm reduction or prevention efforts and has banned MAT entirely (see chapter 6). The revision to MoH Order 200 also constituted a direct slap in the face of European leaders who were financing the Global Fund and pushing the Ukrainian government to enact reforms that met European standards for health care and human rights. The message implicit in the revision of the order was that the Ukrainian state would prioritize its own citizens over the whims of foreign organizations, and that it was aligned with Russian values in determining who its citizens meriting government protections truly were.

The Internet Part of Ukraine, by contrast, picked up on different Putin-esque methodologies for managing internal threats. When the Russian public blamed Chechens for the explosions that shook several major cities in 1999, Putin took to the airwaves and vowed to "rub them [the terrorists] out in the outhouse"—displaying a new level of vulgarity and violence in the authority of the presidential office (Gessen 2017). Thus, to the degree that the state "rubbing out" domestic enemies for the protection of the public was a conceivable action in the years following Putin's remarks, this is precisely what the Internet Party of Ukraine set out to accomplish, and what its public audiences cheered them on for doing. By engaging in the (sometimes violent) social rejection of people who use drugs through public attacks, Internet Party activists carry out their own perceived obligations to marginalize dangerous individuals for the sake of "normal" society. Their protests also highlight the government's failure to uphold its end of this social contract by failing to guarantee the allegiance of police forces and other state actors in this campaign against people who use drugs for the sake of social welfare.

In each case, the "addiction imaginary" provided a robust category of "Otherness" that could be successfully leveraged to voice political values and lay claim to specific arrangements of statehood and sovereignty. As a boundary object, the idea of *narkomany* residing in Ukraine could be taken up by all three actors engaged in these political discourses: the Alliance, the MoH, and the Internet Party of Ukraine. Each was able to talk about, characterize, and make certain claims about this group. Yet, despite the ability this boundary object imparts to conducting a coherent conversation, all participants are reinforcing their own understanding of what the "addiction imaginary" is and how it reflects the ideal relationship between the state and its citizens in everyday life.

Identity and the Addiction Imaginary

In his highly influential book, *Stigma*, sociologist Erving Goffman penned what has become a foundational definition of that very word: "An attribute that makes [the stigmatized] different from others," discrediting someone as "a less desirable kind . . . [as] a person who is bad or dangerous or weak" (Goffman 1963, 3). In their analysis of social stigma against people who use drugs in American culture, Merrill Singer and J. Bryan Page have argued that the imagined "less desirable differences" between people who do and do not use drugs can be very useful (Singer and Page 2014). Among other things, they note that people who use drugs "are a convenient scapegoat when things of various sorts go wrong" (2014, 217) and are often forced to "pay a cost so that some might benefit from [the creation of] a pariah group" (2014, 24). Although stigma is, by definition, a direct and straightforward form of social exclusion, the ways in which value can be extracted from the social imagination of the stigmatized—or, in Singer and Page's words, "the uses of the useless"—are diverse.

Contention over the correct institutional or ideological arrangement in which the state and its citizens should be oriented to one another has long been tethered to questions of health and health care. Political theorists such as Karl Marx, John Locke, and Alexis de Tocqueville have all argued that the health of the population, in one way or another, reflects *how*—in addition to *how well*—a nation-state is functioning. In making these connections, questions about whose health merits protection and how that protection should look strike at the heart of national identity and sovereign authority over that nation. Local views about the territorial and demographic boundaries of the state, the criteria for claiming citizenship, and the obligations of both individual and institutional actors toward each other all collectively form the substrate of national identity. The perception of "the useless," therefore, can have far-reaching effects within the societies that maintain their exclusion. They help define the ideologies and practices through which individual citizens come to understand who they are and where they belong in society.

In this chapter, I have argued that a multi-faceted "addiction imaginary" provides politically engaged actors in Ukraine with a diverse pallet of narrative tropes for articulating values of citizenship, sovereignty, and how an appropriate relationship between citizen and state should look. In the examples detailed above, both the Alliance (an institutional actor with ties to international governance technologies) and the Internet Party of Ukraine (a grassroots organization of protest artists) levied claims against the Ukrainian government, criticizing the leadership for failing to uphold their basic obligations to the citizen population. However, as the Alliance urged government leaders to align their actions with international standards, the Internet Party compelled the government to act upon—and even formalize—the common Ukrainian view that people who use drugs are threats to public order and should be removed from society. Clearly, the latter perspective continues to hold significant sway in the popular imagination.

Together, these examples reveal the plasticity of the "addiction imaginary" in Ukraine and its utility as a discursive tool for defining the limits of the sovereign state and the citizenry it serves. They also reveal the degree to which the medicalization of substance use disorder can scaffold preexisting discourses that selectively marginalize people who use drugs. Even though medicalization often removes moral overtones from mental health symptoms by framing these problems as a disease rather than a personal fault or weakness, the Alliance's appeals to biomedical understandings of substance use disorder did not accomplish this. Instead, it resonated with an "addiction imaginary" that frames *narkomany* as a stigmatized social class—the same object definition of people who use drugs that was defended by the Internet Party of Ukraine. Rather than removing the moral stigma surrounding behavior, the Alliance's attempts to medicalize substance use disorder may have helped social and political leaders draw a clearer, scientifically defined boundary around those parts of society considered to be malignant. They may thus be facilitating the same efforts of containment that were in play before the international global health complex brought MAT to Ukraine, but with greater force and demographic precision.

Chapter 5

The Drugs of Revolution

As we walked to the edge of the park, seeking a quiet place to talk, Alyona lifted up her shirt. She pulled it high over her ribs to show me the swirling scar that wrapped around her belly. It is an indelible mark of the life she has lived and the choices she has made. "Jenny," she said to me matter-of-factly, "I know you are here to learn these stories, to understand the stories of people who are here and using drugs, to know about the things that brought us here, and I, I am practically the social worker here. I used to be the social worker. This is my job; I perceive it as my job, do you understand? Well, my mother was from Pervomaisk—do you know where this is?" This is how Alyona began her story.

Alyona's first husband used drugs for most of his life. Alyona did not share his habit. She struggled to coexist with his substance use, but remained fiercely loyal to him in spite of the difficulties it caused. When he was still quite young, he developed sepsis, likely caused by unsafe injection practices, and suddenly died. Soon after this first tragedy, Alyona was involved in a terrible car crash that claimed her spleen and gave her the gnarled discoloration on the front of her body. Hurt, alone, and with nowhere else to go, she moved in with her late husband's mother in Moscow. They shared an apartment and began supporting themselves as small-time currency traders in the black market. It was in this world that Alyona was first introduced to heroin. She never injected it, but the drug was prevalent, and she would sometimes smoke it or snort it with friends.

Along with casual drug use, physical trauma remained a regular part of Alyona's life in Moscow. She experienced her first ectopic pregnancy and lost a fallopian tube a year after she arrived. This was followed by numerous unplanned pregnancies and abortions—as many as twenty in the subsequent decade. After a while, Alyona settled in with a steady boyfriend, but he frequently subjected her to relational and economic abuse. He would regularly steal from her and try to conceal his actions. Alyona wanted to leave him, but circumstances always seemed to get in the way. After the sudden death of his grandfather left him with no place to live,[1] he moved in with Alyona and began injecting heroin in their home. Bit by bit, Alyona began injecting with him. Soon, she was injecting every day.

Alyona's life became so fraught that she once again decided to make a clean break. She abruptly stopped using heroin. She got a job, began earning money, and lived an "honest life," one for which she said she "would not have to be ashamed before God." Alyona abstained from opioid use for more than two years until, twelve years after her first ectopic pregnancy, she was diagnosed with a second one. She lost her only remaining fallopian tube and her ability to bear children. Her sister died of throat cancer around the same time, and Alyona plunged into another destructive spiral. She began injecting a form of methamphetamine called *vint*. "Do you know what it is?" she asked me. "It's a white drug, it's worse than cocaine. It made me crazy; I was going crazy. Taking all that *vint*, I caught HIV."

As she approached her breaking point, Alyona says her "mother-in-law" began encouraging her to seek treatment:

> "Look, Alyona," she said to me. "Live. Live your life. God loves you. You have so many good things in your life. You can survive. You can help people. You're a good person . . ." And so I was persuaded to come here [to Kyiv], to this [MAT] program. And to start taking [anti-retroviral therapy for HIV]. Before I came here, so many of my friends and boyfriends ended up in jail, and I thought to myself, Alyona, you're going the wrong way. So I moved back to

my [biological] mother's place in this neighborhood and started this MAT. And now I've been coming for four years.

At the time of our meeting, Alyona was ambivalent about her situation. She was happy to have removed the drama in her daily life. She was dating a new man whom she described as "kind, good, and hardworking." He was also a patient at the clinic, and Alyona was incredibly proud of him. At the same time, Alyona struggled to find stable work in Kyiv; she was unable to build a social network that was not bound by the geography of the clinic; and she longed to create the nuclear family she'd never had.

Alyona's story is replete with a kind of dispossession unique to Soviet (and often post-Soviet) society. Caroline Humphrey has argued that the post-Soviet dispossessed "are people who have been deprived of property, work, entitlements . . . people who are themselves no longer possessed. That is, they are no longer inside the quasi-feudal corporations, the collective 'domains' which confer social status on their members" (2002, 21). Common examples of such dispossessed/unpossessed people include "the unemployed; economic migrants; demobilized soldiers, abandoned pensioners, invalids, and single parent families; vagrants and the homeless; and people living in various illegal ways, such as contract laborers without residence permits in large cities [*limitchiki*]" (2002, 21). Those who use drugs (*narkomany*) certainly belong on that list as well.

Most MAT patients in Ukraine, like Alyona, fit Humphrey's description of dispossession in myriad ways. Most are unemployed. Those who do work hold low-paying, dead-end jobs: they are trash collectors, day laborers, and parking lot attendants. Most live with a relative of some kind, often a parent, but lack updated registration paperwork (Ukr: *propyska*), leaving them with no legal claim over their family's property. The death of a family member with whom they live can quickly leave them homeless, as the state will absorb the property and resell it on the public market in the absence of anyone with a valid legal claim, regardless of relation. Furthermore, a significant proportion of MAT patients in Ukraine are coinfected with and actively receiving treatment for HIV and TB (both of which are highly stigmatized). These patients are often associated in the public imagination with vagrancy and the dispossessed underclasses. Most have spent time in prison. Over the course of my research, nearly every MAT patient I met disclosed at least one incident of incarceration or involuntary hospitalization in the past. Once, when I cracked a joke with the staff of the Kyiv clinic about the neverend-ing backgammon games that clients played in the courtyard, a social worker responded, "You know, they've all been in prison at some point. There is nothing to do there but play this game. It's what they're used to."

When viewed through the lens of disposession, a particular irony emerges from Alyona's story. Extraordinary trauma and upheaval (the death of her partner, the head-on collision that claimed her spleen, her ectopic pregnan-cies, her exacerbated substance use disorder, her physically and financially abusive relationships) appear to be the norm, while "normal" elements of life (earning an "honest" living, finding a husband, raising a family) seem extraor-dinary and beyond reach. They have been, for her, practically unattainable. Yet she continually references her desire to build a "normal life" as one of her primary motivations for staying in treatment. It is, by her own account, the primary motivation behind most of her major life decisions.

Making claims to or stating one's desire for a "normal life" is common among Ukraine's MAT patients and among denizens of the post-Soviet sphere in general (Fehérváry 2002; Fournier 2012; Rausing 2014; Yurchak 2008; Zigon 2010). It is an efficient way to position oneself either as morally upstanding within Ukrainian society or, alternatively, as someone econom-ically disadvantaged in relation to residents of wealthier European nations. It's something I heard ordinary people say a lot during my time in Ukraine. The frequency with which the struggle for "normalcy" was invoked by MAT patients in my interviews with them, however, was remarkable. To them a "normal life" carried the promises of reclaiming their lost familial roles and achieving the social integration that had been sacrificed at some point in the past. Few were able to achieve this goal, but everyone receiving MAT seemed to be chasing it.

This is why, several months later, I immediately thought of Alyona when I read an interview with a young woman named Liza Shaposhnik. Ukrai-nian president Viktor Yanukovych had tabled discussions with the EU about an association agreement in the preceding weeks. Many Ukrainians re-sponded with outrage, and the EuroMaidan protests began to take shape in Kyiv's city center. Liza, a volunteer at the protests who had been gaining some local attention, gave an interview to Radio Svoboda, and her words sounded so familiar. "I came to Maidan to stand up for my rights," she said. "The Eu-ropean Union is, for us, a chance to live well, to have a normal life [Rus: *zhit' normal'no*]."

Though central to the EuroMaidan protests, national dialogue that connects European values with a "normal" quality of life first came to a head in Ukraine's 2004 Orange Revolution. Similar to the EuroMaidan revolution, this protest was shorter-lived, immensely influential, and held in the same central square in Kyiv. The Orange Revolution sprang up as a result of Yanukovych's first attempt to claim the Ukrainian presidency. Yanukovych was clearly the favored candidate of Vladimir Putin, a circumcstance that led the public to suspect Kremlin-led foul play when, first, Yanukovych's opponent, Viktor Yushchenko, fell ill from dioxin poison (a toxin produced in very few places on earth, Russia being one of them), and second, when the government-controlled electoral commission announced that Yanukovych had won the election despite exit polls showing him nearly ten points behind (Plokhy 2017). According to political scientist Taras Kuzio, the choice between Yushchenko and Yanukovych was easily framed in the public imagination as a choice between good and evil (Kuzio 2006). Russian-backed candidate Viktor Yanukovych did his best to associate the protests against him with the troublesome "addiction imaginary," calling protestors zombies, cattle, and "drugged" people (Fournier 2012). Some protestors made light of these accusations by carrying syringes with them into the square and displaying them stuck into actual oranges (Durning 2014). The visual pun was meant to be farcical and obvious.

A decade later, from November 2013 to February 2014, the same conscious push away from Soviet social paradigms toward a national community that embraces European values and the "normal life" these values are believed to engender (see Fehérváry 2002) was a central tenet of the EuroMaidan revolution, as was the ridicule of opponents as *narkomany* by the government and protestors alike. Many Ukrainians involved in the protests felt unfairly denied the possibility of living a "normal life" by the country's corrupt leaders and the violence they imposed on the national economy. Liza, who had lived with a physical disability since birth and suffered loss and discrimination as a result, came to embody the public's imagination of its own dispossession at the hands of politicians like Yanukovych. Through the media narrative of Liza's social redemption at EuroMaidan, protestors channeled their own hopes for an end to corruption, an expansion of freedoms, and the achievement of an idyllic and collective "normal life." It is telling, then, that MAT patients so commonly attempt to build a "normal life" for themselves but are almost universally denied acknowledgement or success in these efforts.

The EuroMaidan protests served as a powerful venue in which shared beliefs about community, sovereignty, and personhood could be voiced and amplified. Major narrative events and ideological frames engaged by the charismatic leaders of the revolution helped shape public fervor around the collective project of representing—if not physically enacting—the "true" nation of Ukraine. In this context, Liza was able to achieve what MAT patients typically are not: a right and profitable place in society, characterized by redemption, acceptance, and the accessibility of a celebrated "normal life." In contrast, people who use drugs—and the "addiction imaginary" more broadly—became central elements in EuroMaidan's most oppositional nationalist discourses. Rather than offering opportunities for social redemption, the moral narratives of EuroMaidan actively bolstered the image of people who use drugs as a toxic Other. Throughout the protests, the collective dehumanization of troublesome *narkomany* was clearly (and frequently) articulated, as it helped define true Ukrainianness by representing precisely that undesirable thing that the worthy citizenry was not.

Rehabilitating a Normal Life

Though some MAT patients, including Alyona, disliked certain elements of their medical care, most insisted that they chose to stay on MAT because they had resolved to improve their lives and achieve normalcy. For many, that normalcy meant the fulfillment of the social roles and obligations that had at one point defined them. A woman receiving MAT from a clinic in Odessa described her situation in this way:

> I would like to have a husband . . . I want to prepare my daughter to take care of herself. This is the most important thing: getting your kids on their own two feet. Obviously I want to find a job. Eventually I'd like to have a job. With this [MAT] program, you can find a job, because you just come in the morning to take your pills and then for the rest of the day you are free. You feel fine, just like a normal person. You don't even think all day about needing your next hit, about the money you'd need to score, running around like that. You can . . . I'd like to find a job.

Recall that Lyuda, the young, tropicamide-using mother who received MAT at the same clinic (see chapter 3), offered a similar perspective:

We try to live like normal, healthy people. . . . Here it's just, like, I take my pills and I feel fine. Nothing hurts, I sleep regularly, I eat regularly, and everything's fine. And the whole time your dose is decreasing down to that minimum and then you're already going without and we live like normal people. . . . I can't say that I'm ready because I'm still craving the next high all the time . . . in my head. I struggle with it. I have this daughter who is growing up so fast, and I am very well aware that I need to stop, but it hasn't happened for me.

At first glance, these two statements may appear to reflect very different lived experiences of MAT. The first woman is motivated. She has set concrete goals and sees a clear trajectory for herself through the treatment program. Lyuda, on the other hand, feels stuck. Her words belie a powerful frustration with the program and the way it conflicts with her own physical and emotional impulses. However, these two statements share one key characteristic: both women frame their successes and failures in terms of their ability to engage with their socially proscribed roles as wives and mothers. They, like so many others, use the fulfillment of those roles as a watermark against which to measure not only their progress through treatment but also their legitimacy as members of Ukrainian society.

In interviews, MAT patients staked their claims to "normalcy" along similar axes of social intelligibility, such as professional identity or family identity. Work and the ability to earn an "honest" living were among the most commonly cited elements of the normal personhood MAT patients sought. When I asked how they had felt since starting treatment, many would exclaim that they felt great, normal, so normal that they could find work. One man receiving MAT in Odessa cried "Excellent! [I feel] excellent all day. . . . And, normally, you can even work, and physically work." Some would express dissatisfaction with the program, wishing that the hours were more flexible, that methadone was easier to obtain by prescription. Yet many concluded for themselves that being in the program was better than nothing due in large part to their newfound ability to hold a steady job. "How do I feel in the program?" a young man on MAT in Sevastopol told me. "Alright." He shrugged. He nodded. "I'm working."

In the fall of 2012, I spoke with Vova and Masha, married MAT patients from Simferopol who had come to their clinic with their young baby in tow, about how substance use had prevented them from working or holding down long-term jobs. "When you're on that garbage on the street," Vova told me, "it's not possible to work normally. Because, well, I was working and at the same time I was constantly missing work because I had to manage my [withdrawal symptoms]." As he recounted his story, his wife Masha paced in slow, lazy circles around him, rocking their restless baby to sleep. As she listened, she became upset with his use of street slang. "Speak like a normal person!" she scolded, expressing her strong distaste for these reminders of the life they had left behind. For her, "normal" meant not only becoming a professional person but acting and speaking like one as well.

Some MAT patients took a different approach to their relationship with "normal" employment. Rather than framing MAT as a tool that gave them the ability to work "like normal people," they described the clinical rules and regulations of MAT as the primary obstacle between them and the steady employment they would otherwise achieve. Yulia, woman who received methadone from a clinic in L'viv, described her predicament as follows:

> The way work is here in Ukraine, no one will let you come in at half past ten [most MAT clinics open at 10:00 A.M.]. There's no employer who offers such work. . . . And if I'm not working, how do I manage? What's left for me? To steal? What else? What else remains for me to do? Unless I have a disability, but our disability support doesn't compare to yours. It only gives UAH 800 [about USD 100 at the time of the interview, less than USD 40 at the time of writing] for you to figure out how to live each month. I've got prescriptions that cost more than UAH 800. How do I pay for my house, or support my parents, buy clothes—what do I eat? Do you understand? And so, how is it, being on therapy? Handing it out [by prescription instead of daily dosing at the clinic] would have been better. I would imagine that I could find a job then. . . . I imagine that I would be able to drink liquid methadone at 9:00 A.M., at home, and then go out and head to work. I would be able to get a job. Because not every employer considers people with HIV to be "normal." And as for people in MAT, well, it's a problem.

This woman's testimony differs from that of Masha and Vova in that she voiced displeasure with the structural effect the MAT program has had on her life. However, the meaning she attributed to regular employment is the same as that communicated by others in treatment: "normal" people have jobs, so having a job helps to make you a "normal" person, and the value of MAT care can be measured by the degree of help or hindrance it offers in this regard.

The fulfillment of familial roles was also a major theme in MAT patients' descriptions of the "normal life" they sought to attain. "That's why we come here," another woman from the MAT clinic in Odessa explained, "[People want] to get away from the life of disease. In order not to go to jail, so as not to wake up in wrangling with the law, to live a normal life with their families, with their children, which they finally want to have at that age, middle-aged when they've finally realized." Many patients mentioned their children as a motivation for seeking treatment and acknowledged that MAT provided them with the time they needed to be parents, to actively raise their children. Masha and Vova cite their infant daughter as the anchor holding their new life together. "We have this great joy now," Vova said, gesturing toward his baby. "There is no going back. We have a reason to build a life."

Many MAT patients drew direct connections between the enactment of these social roles (as members of the workforce, as capable parents, as reliable spouses) and their successful integration into broader society. They hoped these roles would put them on the right side of the ideologies that had stigmatized them and relegated them to the social margins. When I asked what he wanted out of the program, Igor, another young man from the Simferopol clinic replied:

> I'd like to rejoin normal society, to not feel like an outcast, to feel like a normal person. To work. Right now, I'm not working, and I feel like, for example, my father is really ill right now. I'd want to help him, but I have no way to help him. I want to help him buy some medications, but he needs an MRI, and that costs UAH 950 [USD 120 at the time of research; USD 47 at the time of writing]. Very few people can afford it.

Vova echoed a similar sentiment. "We [Masha and I] just wanted to come back to life, to normal life, where there is work and a car and everything is fine."

When MAT is used in this way, used by patients to position themselves as more active, "successful" social agents, treatment serves as a technology of the self. Specifically, patients' claims to "normal" personhood are shaped by their tenacious insistence that they are *deserving* of "normal" personhood, that they desire to be welcomed and acknowledged as such. In other cultural settings, treatment for substance use disorder may be wielded by patients and providers in order to excavate a true inner self believed to exist beneath the "addict's" pathological denial (Carr 2010), provide a crutch for the patient's personal agency, weakened by the perpetual impulse to use (Raikhel 2013), or even forge an entirely new subjectivity, remaking the "addict" into a new kind of person with a new set of social dispositions (Zigon 2010). Ukrainian MAT patients, however, do not describe the personhood they wish to embody as obscured by psychological pathology or in the process of formation, as these scholars have observed elsewhere. Rather, they describe the personhood they seek as an element already fully formed within them, which they are unable to fulfill due to the burdens that substance use has put upon them and their relationships. What they seek is better social integration, and that integration is, in common estimation, initially enabled by MAT, which provides them with free time and routine; however, the practical limitations of the program become obstacles once they have regained access to their desired social roles.

Yet, despite these challenges, many MAT patients held onto the hope of social redemption—not just for their own good but for the good of society at large. "Socialization—do you know what it is?" Tamara asked me one day, and replied to her own question:

> It is your infusion into society. If you work, you will somehow cling to normal people. You're not cooking up this garbage with a bunch of other "addicts" [Rus: *s narkomanami*]. Your interests, when you take this pill in this office [MAT], they will diverge dramatically. For the state—this is profitable for the state. Not because the Global Fund pays for the pills, but because they want their citizens to be on the right path. They help us because we have to move towards Europe. You can't have a European country without these programs.

In her mind, and in the mind of many other public health professionals in Ukraine, MAT offers social redemption not only to patients but to the whole state—a state that once left its drug-using citizens behind.

The *Khoziaistvo*

The stories that MAT patients craft about what they want and how they understand treatment to enable or inhibit the realization of those goals are intimately linked with a particular, locally meaningful conception of the social subject. Specifically, the mode of social integration that is sought by MAT patients is grounded in a form of collective personhood forged by late Soviet and early post-Soviet economic realities. This subjectivity has been described as a "dividual" person. In the words of Elizabeth Dunn, a "dividual" person is someone who "acts on the world by acting on others" (Dunn 2004, 126). Though the "dividual" person can manifest in myriad ways, one classic "dividual" practice is a heavy reliance on the secondary markets and systems of exchange that proliferated during the Soviet Union's economies of deficit. These secondary economies included many forms of informal, mutual cooperation such as food sharing between friends, gift swapping among coworkers, and factory managers cutting deals under the table for the redistribution of raw materials (Dunn 2004; Ledeneva 2006; Patico 2008). Maintaining these networks of mutual dependency was an essential practice for those who sought to live a "normal life" during the Soviet era; it was necessary in order to thrive within the structures maintained by the dominant sociopolitical ideology. Put another way, mutually dependent, "dividual" people were considered "normal" because contemporary social structures benefited people who were mutually dependent in this way.

These systems of informal linkages also defined individuals in relation to the state in a normative sense. Katherine Verdery describes this relation as one of "socialist paternalism," a political ethic that "posited a moral tie linking subjects with the state through their rights to a share in the redistributed social product" (1996, 63). According to Caroline Humphrey, this form of sociopolitical order was articulated through the active personification of power. "Crucially," Humphrey observes, "this idea is also represented in the term for state (*gosudarstvo*) deriving from *gosudar* (the sovereign)" (2002, 28). The state, both in the geographic and in the sociopolitical senses, was conceptually rendered as the domain (*khoziaistvo*) of the personified sovereign that brought all its citizens into relation with one another. The personality cult of leadership that defined so much of Soviet politics has not survived into contemporary politics—or, at least, the form that has survived has changed so much that it is not exactly the same phenomenon; however, concepts of cultural heritage (the imperative to "be Ukrainian" in the cultural sense) or even nationalism (the unifying factor of "being Ukrainian" in a political sense) provide convenient stand-ins for mobilizing the discourse of the collective social *khoziaistvo* today.

The concept of *khoziaistvo* dominated the biopolitics of the Soviet period. It defined not only the society that was governed but also an assemblage of administrative controls that were employed to do the work of governing. Instructively, Stephen Collier has identified two constitutive elements of the *khoziaistvo* as a way to imagine society as a collective. The first was "the displacement of the *khoziaistvo*—the nexus of need fulfillment—from the family to the city" during Soviet planning (2011, 83). This meant establishing systems of mutual dependencies both at the administrative level and in the minds of the subject-citizens. The second constitutive move was "the articulation of the city *khoziaistvo* by prescriptive, substantive norms that encoded human needs into 'complexes' of elements that could be plugged into plans" (2011, 83). The agents who produced these administrative plans under the Soviet regime considered the region as a whole, rather than a collection of distinct regional enterprises that could be managed individually. Thus, the discourse of the people's domain (Rus: *narodnoe khoziaistvo*) or the single national economy and national identity were crafted, one that Collier has aptly called "a mono-society" (2011, 74).

The structures and norms that were used to encode human needs for Soviet administrative powers resonate with the claims made by MAT patients about who "normal" people are and what "normal" people do. These norms are also apparent in clinicians' assertions about the degree to which their patients want (or don't want) to "get better" while they are in treatment (see chapter 3). Each of these contemporary discourses seen in the MAT clinic levy moral claims about the ability of people who use drugs to forge the appropriate forms of mutual interdependence constitutive of *khoziaistvo*. They are assertions about the capacity of people who use drugs to achieve "infusion into society," as Tamara so aptly described, through which they would be able not only to become "normal people" but to "*cling* to [other] normal people" as well.

The key point here is that MAT patients do not simply aim to achieve some generalized, broad-stroke ideal of social integration for themselves; rather, they are aiming to achieve the *only* form of social integration permitted within the monocultural discourse of *khoziaistvo*. Furthermore, admission into the *khoziaistvo* is not a stepwise process. One's insider/outsider status is binary. This social reality affected even my own experiences in Ukraine, as well as those of the other foreign researchers who made up my primary academic community while I was conducting my research.[2] While attempting to navigate our own entrées into Ukrainian professional and social circles, many of us would reassure ourselves by repeating the mantra—shared from researcher to researcher—that "until you're in, you're out."[3] We found comfort in the phrase's implicit message that social acceptance tended to happen all at once, that the feeling of spinning one's wheels was not necessarily a sign of failure but rather a symptom of the first phase of ethnographic research in this part of the world. I contend that this awareness, considered wisdom in my academic circles, is a basic principle known to Ukrainian citizens who were born and raised in a society that is given discursive shape by the concept of *khoziaistvo*. This is why MAT patients' claims to normalcy, or to their desire to be "normal," continue despite the appearance that they are stuck in their marginalized positions.

The Heroine of Maidan

Unfortunately, Ukrainians with a history of substance use, even those in treatment, are rarely able to make this transition from "out" to "in." The cause of this consistent failure can be discerned by taking a closer look at the case of Liza Shaposhnik, who *did* successfully end her own dispossession and move from outside of the Ukrainian *khoziaistvo* to within. She stood out among the other volunteers in the EuroMaidan kitchens and quickly became well-known both for her efforts in the antigovernment movement and her embodiment of traditional Ukrainian gender roles. The mechanisms that maintained Liza's marginalization are quite similar to those that marginalize people who use drugs. In this way, the beginnings of their stories are also quite similar. However, at the points where their paths diverge, a potent ethopolitics (Rose 2007) can be discerned—a moral reckoning and social policing of individuals' inner psychological states.

The popular narrative of Liza Shaposhnik, which was covered in Russian- and Ukrainian-language media (Bereza 2013; Gorskaya 2013, 2015; Makar 2014), in English-language media (Shevchenko 2014), and even picked up by Reuters (2013), goes something like this. She was born in Siberia, the daughter of a Russian mother and a Ukrainian father. Her parents relocated to Odessa when she was young, and she spent most of her childhood there. Liza was born with cerebral palsy, and she suffered frequent teasing from other children. Eventually, she found relief from the stigma in adolescence when she moved to a special boarding school. As a young adult, Liza relocated again to the Donets'k region of Ukraine where she was able to rent a room in a hostel and support herself as a fruit vendor. Finally, in September 2013, Liza made her final move to Kyiv in the hopes of improving her situation. She rented her own apartment and again began working as a vendor.

Two months after she arrived in the capital city, the EuroMaidan movement began to take shape in Kyiv's central square, the eponymous Maidan Nezalezhnosti (Independence Square). Liza learned that activists were protesting the president's suspension of an association agreement with the EU and decided to join the efforts (Gorskaya 2013). She was on the main square the night of November 30, 2013, when a heavily armed faction of the national police, the Berkut, stormed the area and violently attacked student protesters. Liza's story from this night is dramatic and harrowing. She recalled sliding down the glass-paneled roof of the Globus mall, a steep, two-story incline fixed into a hill on the edge of the square, to escape the Berkut's truncheons and flee to safety. Fortunately, she was able to evade police forces without injury (Bereza 2013). Her presence during this terrible event, which became a major turning point in the protests, afforded her narrative no small amount of legitimacy in the eyes of other Kyiv residents. Following this attack, the scope of the Euro-Maidan protests grew dramatically. Tens of thousands of Ukrainians took to the streets to reject the violence displayed on November 30 and to demand the resignation of President Viktor Yanukovych.

Liza then learned that volunteers were being recruited to assist with the management of this new popular enterprise and she reported to the kitchens to see if there was something she could do. She was at first tasked with carrying trays of sandwiches to protesters in the square. Liza has limited physical mobility in her hands, so this job turned out to be quite challenging. She switched roles a few times after that. For a short while, she sliced lemons for tea and garnish. Eventually, she settled into a permanent post: she sat at a table every day tearing the tags off of tea bags, which kept the tags from tangling and cups of tea from spilling as they were distributed on the square. Liza's hard work and dedication inspired such affection from her coworkers that they decided to name the kitchens of EuroMaidan in her honor (Gorskaya 2013).

The contribution of these kitchens to the revolution, in general, was largely symbolic. Though many who chose to occupy the square day in and day out

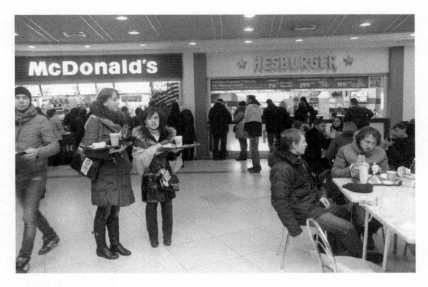

EuroMaidan demonstrators gather in the food court of the Globus shopping mall for a meal.
Photo by author.

relied on food and supplies brought in from the outside, the vast majority of protestors stopped by the square only during weekend rallies or in the evenings after work. They could eat at home whenever they pleased. Besides that, the Globus shopping center, a luxury mall that was built underground in Kyiv's city center, remained open during the protests. One could take an escalator down from inside the barricaded square into the mall's food court and buy a pizza or a hamburger at any time. The protestors with whom I spoke, however, felt a deep appreciation for the modest soups and canapés that were served from the kitchens. These foods fostered a strong atmosphere of solidarity and mutual assistance—of collective "dividuality."

Thus, despite the arguably modest value of her work product, her role as a tea bag organizer generated great satisfaction from other volunteers who saw just as much, if not more, value in her *having* a job to do than in the deliverable results that this job produced. Liza was valued not simply for her labor, but for the fact that she *wanted* to work, for the fact that she selflessly offered her time and energies without being told to do so. This marks the first time that Liza succeeded where MAT patients often fail. She embodied the habitus of a "normal" person, achieving symbolic "normalcy," by first insisting that she contribute to the collective effort, regardless of what product or benefit that work created, and second, by being *allowed to do so*. It was at her tea tag-tearing post, in fact, that the media discovered her and gave her a short burst of celebrity. She was photographed as she sat with a moving box full of tea bags to one side of her and a pile of torn tea tags on the other, working diligently, tirelessly, day after day.

The success of Liza's symbolic "normalcy" during the course of the Euro-Maidan protests can be measured by the public's opinion of her and her disposition. For example, Liza was described by many EuroMaidan partici-pants as humble, as a deserving person who wanted very little for herself. I heard this from friends and strangers alike. Many cited her statement, printed in the newspaper *Ukrainska Pravda*, that she longed only "to see a specialist once in [her] life . . . one who did not purchase their diploma . . . to have ac-cess to a health sanatoria, and to have a free massage" (Bereza 2013) as evi-dence of her humility. For someone who appeared so frail, she asked for very little. A popular website that chronicled the events of EuroMaidan listed Liza as one of the "True Heroes" of the revolution, along with the monk who rang the bells at St. Michael's Cathedral all night during a second Berkut raid on December 11; the metro driver who, with horror, announced those same police attacks against protesters to metro passengers as they were taking place; and two pensioners from Ivano-Frankivsk who spent their entire sav-ings on a bus rental for transporting local residents to Kyiv to join the pro-tests. On this website, Liza is quoted as saying "I never imagined that I could be a needed and useful person. It's like I've been born again—not sick but healthy" (Inspired.com.ua 2014).

The narrative into which Liza's story was woven reached its final denoue-ment in May 2014 when she married fellow EuroMaidan activist Vitaly Popov. On her head, she wore a crown of flowers—on her torso, brightly col-ored *vyshyvanky* (shirts decorated with traditional Ukrainian embroidery patterns). On her legs, she wore military fatigues and sturdy combat boots. Liza and Vitaly, along with a five-piece band and several armed militia mem-bers, were paraded down Kyiv's main boulevard, Khreshatyk, from the central square to Kyiv City Hall atop an armored tank provided by Pravyi Sektor, a radical-nationalist group that played a major role in organizing de-fense forces for the protest camp. After the ceremony, the entourage cara-vanned down Shevchenko Boulevard then made a stop at the memorials for the protestors who were killed by the police in late February on Institutska St. There, the newlywed couple stopped to speak with reporters and showed off their wedding rings. Their matching bands were molded to resemble rubber car tires, the likes of which were burned by protesters along the barricades in the weeks prior (Makar 2014).

Liza was a beautiful flash in the pan of public interest, because she reflected many of the hopes and ambitions of EuroMaidan protestors. Her story is one of personal redemption, but it is also a story of biopolitical redemption. She overcame disability, oppression, even a "backward" thinking family, as the story goes, to build an independent life for herself and contribute to an important social cause. She was viewed as "deserving," "humble," "the most important drop of water in the ocean [of revolutionaries]" ("Liza Shaposhnik" n.d.). Liza became a local hero because, despite the odds, she achieved social acceptance and integration. Also despite the odds, she achieved the status of a married woman, finding deliverance from her former life of exclusion in this ultimate fulfillment of her gendered role as a Ukrainian woman. Liza became an icon for what Marian Rubchak called a return to "real Ukrainian-ness," a phenomenon accomplished by means of women birthing and raising "real" Ukrainians (1996, 318). This is the second point at which Liza succeeded where MAT patients often fail. As a married woman, Liza could not only be a part of the true *khoziaistvo*; she could also productively contribute to it, putting her successful social integration to work for the good of the country, the good of the collective.

Liza was beloved because she overcame powerful obstacles to achieve not simply a life, but that fantasy-like "normal life" that was positioned at the center of the public's collective imagination—one of work, marriage, community, and home. Liza also displayed the outward characteristics of someone legitimately seeking social redemption—or "infusion into society." Her actions reflected her desire, her will, to take on appropriate social roles. Thus, her efforts to engage in systems of mutual dependency (slicing lemons, removing tea tags) were valued far beyond the practical contribution of her work, and her advancement at the end of the protests to the status of a wife and potential mother was enthusiastically welcomed by those around her precisely because of that contribution. And though Liza worked for the sake of the revolution, and though MAT patients so often sought a paying job (wage labor) for the sake of their families (arguably a different kind of work), both sought opportunities to perform labor of some kind for the sake of their social connections. Igor in Simferopol sought money for his father's surgery. Yulia in L'viv hoped to support her parents. Liza and MAT patients alike sought work to deepen their infusion into their social relationships, but only Liza was celebrated with a parade through town.

Slavery, Agency, and Social Exclusion

It was deeply ironic, then, that MAT patients, who clearly harbored the same goals and values as many of those who gathered in the city center to protest government corruption, were not simply relegated to the margins of the revolution, but were explicitly prevented from entering the protest camps. Signage and verbal instructions from guards at EuroMaidan's gates made it clear that neither drugs nor the individuals who used them were welcome in the official space of the revolution. This is because these protests made manifest a particular form of social exclusion that coexists with the social imaginary of the *khoziaistvo*. Through a collective assessment of the internal states of people who use drugs and of the degree to which they are able to think freely (or not), a clear determination is made as to whether such individuals can be integrated into society to join the collective of "dividual" citizens. This is a kind of ethopolitics (Rose 2007), a system of social distinction that discriminates between individuals according to their perceived mental freedom, their ability to act as agents of their own will. Those welcomed into the *khoziaistvo*, like Liza, are considered to be independent thinkers. They act with moral correctness and do so of their own volition. Those who are excluded, on the other hand, are believed to lack personal will. They do not possess the free-thinking abilities of truly independent social agents. In this way, the concept of the *khoziaistvo* dovetails with the way in which contemporary "addiction imaginaries" in Ukraine deny people who use drugs—whether or not they are in treatment—any such claims to personal agency.

The political discourse in and around the EuroMaidan revolution produced many examples of these concepts in action. For instance, the denial of others' personal agency was used in many smear campaigns against opposing political factions. Fittingly, drug use was a common trope in such attacks. Many reports of drug use at EuroMaidan surfaced in Kremlin-controlled Russian media. One exemplary piece, published by *Voice of Russia*, recounted an apocryphal story of a young couple from Kyiv who went to EuroMaidan to be revolutionaries. While inside the barricades, the two youngsters allegedly called friends and described the powerful emotions and euphoric atmosphere that surrounded them. Shortly after leaving the protest camps, the girl began to experience strange symptoms including headaches, nausea, and high blood pressure. Her boyfriend fell ill with a similar malady soon after. They went to a hospital for treatment and were told by the medical staff they were suffering withdrawal from synthetic drugs—drugs that had, according to the article, been secretly fed to them through the soups, teas, and other foodstuffs produced in the EuroMaidan kitchens. The same *Voice of Russia* article also appealed to the allegedly drugged state of the EuroMaidan protesters to explain the violence that erupted February 18–20, 2014, when nearly one hundred protesters were killed by police violence. Viktor Ivanov, then head of the Russian Federal Drug Control Service, was quoted saying that "participants in the Maidan riot were under the influence of drugs, which resulted in 'an absolutely abnormal psychoactive condition'" (*Voice of Russia* 2014).

Attempts made during EuroMaidan to deny the personal agency or responsibility of others extended beyond the realm of drug use, as well. Anti-Maidan activists (progovernment protestors who rallied in a different, nearby public park) were also subjected to agency-denying rhetoric. According to EuroMaidan protesters with whom I spoke, anti-Maidan protesters represented a government that did not serve them and protested willingly for meager cash payments from government officials. EuroMaidan activists perceived them as weak in conscience, weak in spirit, willing to sacrifice their principles for the smallest advantage. I heard them called cattle. I heard them called slaves and prostitutes. I even heard the portmanteau "prostitushky" (a dual reference to "selling oneself" and to *titushky*, a name used to refer to hired government thugs) used disparagingly against them. Similar epithets were launched against the Ukrainian police officers who lashed out at protesters. Those people were brainwashed. They were zombies. They were animals, not even human. All "opponents" of the EuroMaidan movement were characterized similarly: as weak in moral constitution, willing to surrender their human values for small, short term gains, brainwashed or brain damaged, incapable of acting like humans, or, worst of all, not even human to begin with.

These discourses of distinction are older than the EuroMaidan revolution. They were prevalent during Ukraine's Orange Revolution in 2004, as well. At the height of these protests, signs could be seen around the Maidan that read, "We are not slaves." Anthropologist Anna Fournier interviewed a

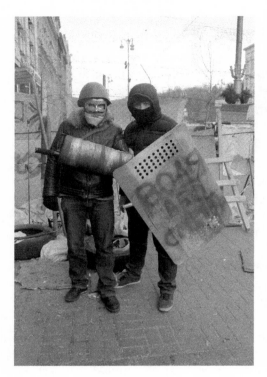

EuroMaidan demonstrators sport home-made protective gear. One holds a riot shield that reads "Volia abo Smert'," which can be translated from Ukrainian as "Liberty or death." The word "volia" can also be taken to mean "free will," rendering the meaning of this phrase ideologically specific but syntactically ambiguous. Photo by author.

middle-aged political science professor at the Orange Revolution who elaborated on what this phrase meant: "What are slaves? A silent, amorphous mass. Slaves carry out the tasks [*vykonuiut zavdannia*] given to them, otherwise they know their heads will be cut off. Slaves are mute, but now, now we can already talk. We have freedom [*volia*]" (2012, 146). Put another way, "slaves" are perceived to be people who lack the will to act as citizen-subjects. To the degree that "addiction imaginaries" reflect local theories of subjectivity and volition, one could say that "slaves" and *narkomany* are generally the same kind of people. They differ only in that *narkomany* reveal their deficiency of will through substance use. "Slaves" may not present themselves so obviously. The interchangeability of these terms, however, makes sense if the goal of using them is to dehumanize and to strip those accused of being "drugged" or "slaves" of the capacity for agency.

Protestors in the Orange Revolution used terms like "slaves" and "cattle" to describe both those who opposed the protests and those who chose not to

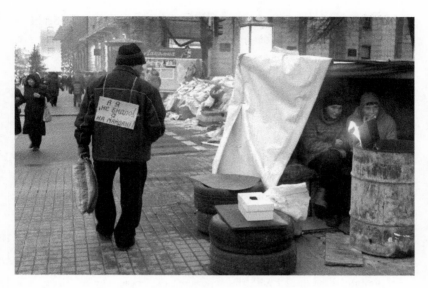

A man walks through the EuroMaidan protest camp wearing a sign that reads "Because I am not cattle, I am at the Maidan!" (Ukr: *A ya ne bydlo! Ya na Maidani!*). Photo by author.

be involved. The supporters of presidential candidate Viktor Yushchenko, the opposition leader around whom the Orange Revolution protesters rallied, claimed that counterprotesters who backed the Kremlin-endorsed candidate Viktor Yanukovych (the same president EuroMaidan protestors opposed in 2013 and 2014) were coming out "because they had been paid to attend" or had been "zombified [*zombirovanni*] brainwashed, or drugged" (Fournier 2012, 8). Many students defied parents and teachers by becoming active participants in the 2004 revolution, disparaging those who did not do the same. One student explained, "99 percent of people in our country are *bydlo* [lit. cattle, but meaning in this context, ignorant and destitute], they have no money, they don't know *anything*" (Fournier 2012, 86).

The discursive history of exclusion at these two protests reveals that those individuals outside the *khoziaistvo* are perceived in popular culture as quintessential examples of this kind of apolitical, asocial, zombielike individual, hopelessly lost to their wanton impulses. MAT patients, in particular, become articulated in the popular imagination not simply through lay explanatory models of "addiction" but also through these locally salient theories of social subjectivity. Recall, again, the complaint of the nurse in the TB hospital (see chapter 3) that her patients had no will to be involved in their own health or the lives of anyone else. "Doctors tell them to come here [to this office to receive anti-TB pills], but they just hang out, they talk in the hallway, and then they leave. They are alcoholics, 'addicts' [Rus: *alkogoliki, narkomany*]. They have no desire. Maybe the wife already died, the daughter is already sick. It's all the same to them. . . . That's 'addiction' [Rus: *narkomaniia*]." One could replace the word "addiction" in this comment with "slavery," "zombies," or "brainwashing" and render this complaint applicable to Berkut officers, government-paid thugs, or anti-Maidan activists.

Though this mechanism of social exclusion is pervasive in contemporary Ukraine, the story of Liza Shaposhnik's revolutionary heroism in EuroMaidan's kitchens is evidence that exclusion from the *khoziaistvo* can be overcome—at least temporarily. This might lead one to think that people who use drugs should, in principle, be able to overcome this obstacle as well. This seems especially true given that Liza's formal status as a member of the group of people with disabilities is parallel with the experience of people who use drugs who are in treatment in a number of key ways. Both groups are officially registered and classified as known entities to the state. Both conditions—disability and substance use disorder—are subject to intense social othering, fueled by the stigma attached to the outward appearance of bodily pathologies. Even more important, both groups face significant limitations in their ability to find profitable work. People who use drugs are limited by the physical practicalities of their chemical dependency: many of the least stable find themselves forced to direct much of their time and attention toward the daily "hunt" for drugs in order to avoid withdrawal. Those with officially recognized disabilities are given a meager amount of social security to live on each month, but in exchange, are prohibited from participating in the formal job market.[4] Many, like Liza, are able to find low-wage jobs that pay under the table, but the vast majority of occupations remain inaccessible.

Exclusion from the formal job market complicates the social intelligibility of opioid-dependent people and those with disabilities alike. The Soviet idea that one's social identity is directly linked to one's labor toward the collective enterprise remains one of this era's most potent ideological legacies. As political scientist Mary Hawkesworth has observed, "The social significance of a person . . . the criterion of value of a person lies in his/her relation to work, in the socially useful work of the individual" (1980, 72: cited in Fournier 2012, 20). This explains Liza's ability to overcome social exclusion by simply performing work rather than producing a work product of meaningful value. However, a major difference lies in the fact that Liza's exclusion from the labor force is ultimately out of her control (she did not *choose* to have cerebral palsy), whereas people who use drugs are frequently blamed for creating the situation that effectively removed their ability to work. Discourses of "wanting" as a therapeutic disposition (see chapter 3) situate responsibility for the dispossession of opioid-dependent people onto their own alleged psychological weaknesses.

In keeping with the stereotype that *narkomany* have no desire, no will to be "normal," the intentional refusal to work is deeply ingrained into the popular stereotype of drug and alcohol use (Fournier 2012, 95). This fact is well illustrated by an example from Fournier's ethnography of high school education in Kyiv. One day, a teacher read the following passage from the Soviet constitution aloud for her class: "Article 60: It is the duty of, and a matter of honor for, every able-bodied citizen of the USSR to work conscientiously in his chosen, socially useful occupation, and strictly to observe labor discipline. Evasion of socially useful work is incompatible with the principles of socialist society" (2012, 79). The teacher then observed that citizens' right to work was also guaranteed by the Ukrainian constitution. When a student joked, "Or to not work!" she answered, "Yes, of course, if you want to sit with a bottle [*sydity z pliashkoyu*] all day, you can!" "In this case," Fournier notes, "'sitting with a bottle' means doing nothing or being a 'lazy bum'" (2012, 79). In contrast, Liza was able to fully and successfully embody the symbolic elements of "normalcy" because her work in the EuroMaidan's kitchens could be interpreted as an act of protest against her forced exclusion from work. Liza was perceived not simply as a dedicated member of the revolution, but as the physical personification of individual agency and the desire to exist fully within the collective.

People who use drugs, on the other hand, are viewed as the antithesis of Liza. At EuroMaidan, they were unable to heroically overcome their social exclusion because they were believed to have forged that exclusion on their own. They were also believed to pose a particularly dangerous threat to society. Their alleged mental weaknesses and chemical dependencies are thought to render them vulnerable to psychological exploitation. A cunning enemy could easily fill the crowd at a counterprotest or a unit of government police officers or a brigade of separatist fighters, armed and unwieldy at a militia checkpoint, with such manipulable, zombielike individuals. No matter

what attempts MAT patients made to assert their desire for social integration, to meet their social obligations, or to fulfill their proscribed roles as productive members of society, these efforts remained overwhelmed by a
powerful, circular logic that rendered them less than human in the eyes of
their neighbors. The end result is that people who use drugs find themselves
locked into a place of social exclusion, unable to gain entry to "normal" society so long as any substances, whether from the street or from the MAT
clinic, remain a part of their lives.

We're Staying Here, All of Us

Through both the exclusion of people who use drugs and the beautiful popular narrative of Liza Shaposhnik's social redemption, this chapter has
decoded the social value placed on building a "normal life," on building for
oneself a socially intelligible "dividual" subjectivity. This chapter has also
argued that this "normal life" deviates from the neoliberal ideal in that self-
determination and self-actualization alone are insufficient to build a valid social identity. To achieve a "normal life" in Ukraine today, one must also
contend with a system of social distinction that equates socially acceptable
forms of sobriety and self-sacrifice with spiritual cleanliness and deserved-
ness, rendering those with socially unacceptable behaviors undeserving and
even nonhuman. Over time, these kinds of social distinctions tend to become
naturalized in cultural logics, forming part of the collective habitus of a given
community. Dehumanization produces binary relationships—the human vs.
the nonhuman; citizens vs. zombies; us vs. them. Engagement with these discourses may actively discourage public tolerance for a pluralistic society. At
the very least, these discourses provide easy justification for those who would
discourage social or political tolerance of one kind or another.

Partway through our long conversation about her life in Moscow and then
in Kyiv, Alyona expressed some resentment toward Anton, the official social worker at her Kyiv-based MAT clinic. She was angry that he appeared
so dismissive of the challenges patients faced. She accused him of criticizing
them for not finding work when the clinic's schedule was what prevented
them from working in the first place, and she had unflattering things to say
about his work and his character. "He should be defending us," she said, "but,
you know, he's like that." I wondered how much her assessment of Anton's

work performance was influenced by the fact that *she* had served as the de facto social worker at this clinic before he arrived. Alyona believed her ability to council and guide others to be one of her greatest gifts, and it was clear that she felt very much at home in that role. It gave her a sense of purpose and affirmed the most positive parts of her self-image. Now that she had been displaced from this identity and become just another patient at the clinic, Alyona needed a new opportunity for self-fulfillment. She was once again pursuing the same goals as her peers: work, a purpose, a "normal life."

"I'm a very straightforward person," Alyona told me. "Do you understand what that means? I was a healthy, *normal* person. I always helped everyone, you see. Fate saw to that. Our nurses here say to me 'Alyona, you must have had nine children in a past life. Maybe you had so many kids and now you need to use this life to relax . . .'"

"What do you mean when you say 'normal person'?" I asked. She replied:

Living like normal people? It's like, look, when people don't use drugs, they have something for themselves. They have a purpose in life. Some just want more money. They go crazy over trying to get more money. But there's still something else, you know? Those who seek out drugs, or who want to gather up things, they don't understand that each person has a purpose. Each person must be sincere in their heart and not do harm to anyone, not want harm for anyone. And living your life, being kind to others is the most important thing you can do.

As Humphrey has noted, "The dispossessed make mythicized image signs to the citizenry. . . . We hear an endlessness in the narratives of the dispossessed, in their stories that keep starting up again each time they experience another disappointment or another rebuff" (2002, 33). MAT patients are indeed caught in a recursive loop of social marginalization, stuck in a "blind spot" (Keshavjee 2014) of the Ukrainian health-care and social-services systems. However, the more time I spent in the clinics and hospitals where these individuals are contained, the more I felt as if that blindness was intentionally forged. MAT patients often entered this treatment program in the hopes of achieving greater freedom and social recovery, but they soon found themselves in a place with few options, no exit, nowhere else to move on to. If, as Humphrey suggests, "The narratives of the dispossessed only end when they are no longer dispossessed" (2002, 33), then the stories of MAT patients in Ukraine are fated to carry on unchanged for a very long time.

As Alyona and I rounded the bend in the path and approached the clinic gates, I asked her, "What do you want for the future?"

"To keep coming here for a while," she answered. "I'll be here for a while and I'll slowly lower my dose. I want to be able to work somewhere, to be needed, or helpful."

"Do you ever want to quit the program completely?"

"The folks here, we have no idea what will happen tomorrow. This program is in place [funds have been promised by the Global Fund] until 2017. After that, the AIDS Alliance in Kyiv won't sponsor us anymore, because the government won't offer any funds. . . . We're all staying here, though. All of us."

Chapter 6

SOVEREIGNTY AND ABANDONMENT

But they could not stay—at least, not all of them. In 2014, violent disruption in the Autonomous Republic of Crimea and in the southeastern Donbas region of Ukraine severed the fragile ties connecting many of the country's most vulnerable people to basic medical care. Thousands of lives have been lost due to military conflict and the resultant collapse of institutions upon which many relied. Still more lives were lost, as this chapter details, not by concrete acts of war per se, but by political design. In the context of this geopolitical crisis, the exploitation, abandonment, and extrajudicial killing of socially vulnerable people who use drugs were used as means toward political ends. One of those people was named Dima.

I met Dima in 2012 at a clinic in Simferopol where he received MAT: the same clinic where the physicians Ivan and Pavel worked and cracked jokes about cucumbers (see chapter 2); the same clinic where Masha and Vova came with their baby girl and chatted with Sergey and me about *shirka* and their prospects for employment (see chapter 5). Dima called himself a *narkoman*. When we were first introduced, it had been four full years since he first started MAT in Simferopol and stopped using other drugs. In May 2014, when his clinic shut down, it would have been nearly five and a half.

During one of our interviews, I asked Dima why he entered this MAT program in the first place. "I didn't think much about the bigger picture then," he told me:

> I came here to figure out more immediate problems. I had just met my girl-friend. I was always lying to her, telling her that I had some kind of job to get to. At eight in the evening, when we would be out for a walk, I would need to run off. I'd say I had some kind of job, as an excuse. But, she started to figure out what I was doing. And I thought, I need to get on this program, first of all to save the relationship. First, my family started to suspect, she started to suspect that I was on drugs. And second, things had started to really break down at my work. I would come in for a half a day, leave for my lunch break, and never come back. I realized that I needed something in my life to change somehow, that I needed to start on this program.

He did. Two years later, Dima and his girlfriend were married. They have a baby girl who would be, as I write this, approaching her sixth birthday.

Despite the love Dima had for his family and the happiness they were building together, his life slipped back into chaos when he lost access to his medication in the summer of 2014. Within a day of then-president Viktor Yanukovych fleeing Ukraine under pressures from the EuroMaidan revolution, Russian troops invaded the Crimean peninsula, expelled Ukrainian security forces there, and brought the region under Russian control. Two months later, and with very little notice, Russia shut down all MAT programs in Crimea as part of their efforts to secure political control over the region. The consequences of these closures for MAT patients in Crimea were predictable. The risk of opioid overdose is up to twenty-five times higher than normal immediately following the abrupt cessation of treatment (Davoli et al. 2007). Of the approximately eight hundred people receiving MAT in Crimea at the time of the closures, as many as one hundred died in the subsequent weeks (Kazatchkine 2014). Most suffered a fatal overdose after relapsing into opioid use. Some took their own lives. Dima was among the first to die.

As Russia was exerting control over Crimea, another separatist crisis was also brewing simultaneously in eastern Ukraine. Opposition to the post-EuroMaidan, post-Yanukovych government, which had been growing for several months, finally reached its boiling point when Russian operatives crossed the Ukrainian border and transformed that local fervor into an armed and organized separatist movement. With this, the areas surrounding Donets'k and Luhans'k—two major industrial cities in Ukraine's eastern Donbas region near the Russian border—began moving in the same direction South Ossetia and Transnistria had a decade earlier. Specifically, separatist forces and Russian leaders collaborated to bolster the legitimacy of these breakaway regions as independent states. Much of the Ukrainian public and representatives in the post-EuroMaidan government in Kyiv fought to denounce the leaders of these de facto states as hooligans and frauds. Each group found the vilification—and sometimes abuse and torture—of *narkomany* to be efficient means for projecting these political messages.

Both of these geopolitical crises, the annexation of Crimea and the separatist war in Donbas, are important to this analysis of the "addiction imaginary." As I have argued in this book, the way a state responds to drug use and drug-use-related social problems reveals much about its foundational ideological concepts such as the state, citizenship, and national identity. The "addiction imaginary" has long been fertile ground for the articulation of social values and leveraging claims of political authority, especially during times of rapid social change (Singer and Page 2014). These two geopolitical conflicts are both moments in which discourses of national sovereignty were broken down, altered, and reconstituted around a new, non-Ukrainian national identity. Just as political actors like the Alliance and the Internet Party of Ukraine have lobbied for what they each see as the "correct" relationship between the sovereign state and its citizens, and just as the protestors at Kyiv's EuroMaidan engaged in a collective, protracted statement about where the boundaries of that citizenry should be drawn, so the military and paramilitary forces wresting Crimea and Donbas out of Ukrainian control have used these conflict zones to enact new forms of citizenship, fighting for the inclusion of some and the exclusion of others.

These patterns of inclusion and exclusion are worth investigating because they reflect so much of the ideological foundation that renders these political power grabs possible. Especially when we consider sovereignty not as an abstract confabulation of power but as an "assemblage of administrative strategies" (Ong 2006, 98), it becomes possible to scrutinize the biopolitical logic through which a given sovereign power is enacted by looking at the social policies and structures it seeks to enforce. The sovereign "shock therapy" carried out in Crimea and Donbas relied on the rapid, occasionally jarring reconfiguration of those administrative strategies, and the redefinition of citizenship was a crucial component of these exercises. The systematic denial of basic rights to those deemed "outsiders" in the new sovereign arrangement was key as well. Ethnic minorities were especially vulnerable in this regard. Crimean Tatars (Walker 2016) and Roma communities in the Donbas (Baer 2014) have both experienced systematic oppression following the loss of Ukrainian control. Yet an examination of the most widely circulated discourses reveals a distinct and familiar pattern. All of Ukraine's breakaway and secessionist movements, as well as the pro-Ukrainian citizens who opposed them, focused much of their energy on waging public battle with the same paper tiger: local residents who use drugs.

Ultimately, the enactment of sovereignty over these de facto, non-Ukrainian states hinged upon structural and systematic violence against people who use drugs—sometimes using the very public health programs designed to serve them as a weapon for enacting that violence. For the residents of Crimea and Donbas, these new states would become manifest through the delivery of citizens' entitlements (e.g., pensions, health care, kindergartens) as well as through the enforcement of citizens' obligations (e.g., taxes, registration, civil law). As a group already suffering intense social stigma, people who use drugs were easy prey for state authorities wishing to make public displays of their power through structural, symbolic, and physical violence. Likewise, the "addiction imaginary" has frequently been invoked by leaders and publics in Ukraine, occupied Crimea, and separatist territories in Donbas as they sought to affirm or deny each others' legitimacy as a state. In this way, internationally funded health-care programs for people who use drugs, like MAT, caught in these geopolitical conflicts transformed into something much more than practical systems of health-care delivery; they were ideal sites for enacting the kind of sovereign "shock therapy" that separatist leadership needed to seize power, to redraw the bounds of the citizenry by publicly excising those labeled dangerous and unworthy.

We, Us, Ours

In Soviet rhetoric, the political body of the nation was commonly referred to through the possessive pronoun *svoi*. Though there is no exact equivalent in English, *svoi* can be reasonably well-translated from either Russian or Ukrainian to mean "us" or "ours." *Svoi* is distinct from other possessive pronouns, such as "mine" (*moi*) or "ours" (*nash*) in that it refers back not necessarily to the speaker but to the most recently nominated subject. In this way, *svoi* carries meaning similar to the English modifier "own," as in "her own" or "our own." Anthropologist Aleksei Yurchak has described the social symbolism of *svoi* as "the common sociality of young Soviet people . . . used by most rank-and-file members and secretaries [of Soviet youth organizations] to refer to themselves and their peers, especially when distinguishing themselves" (Yurchak 2008, 103). *Svoi,* then, was used to mean "us," or "we the Soviet people," but in a way that clearly evoked that Soviet notion of social integration and unity without explicitly calling it by name.

Similar to the concept of *khoziaistvo*, which stood for the full assemblage of social, material, and administrative structures out of which the nation was composed, the term *svoi* referenced not only citizenship within that collective but also a specific configuration of citizens' rights and obligations in relation to the state. Those who are *svoi* are privileged with certain rights: rights to education, to safety, to work, and to health. At the same time, those who are *svoi* also have a duty to protect the body politic—as EuroMaidan activists sought to do in the protest camps (see chapter 5), as the Internet Party claimed to do while raiding commercial store fronts in Odessa (see chapter 4). If citizens engaged in deviant or otherwise problematic behavior that brought risk into the community, Yurchak observes, "The ultimate punishment was to be expelled from *svoi*" (2008, 111). An ejection from *svoi* meant being barred from the community's systems of mutual care and responsibility and losing one's sense as a valued, needed, "dividual" person.

Today, in the post-Soviet space, *svoi* can represent many things, from the shared cultural and historical legacies that unite this part of the world to the fine lines of distinction between class, ethnicity, and nationality that people of Eastern Europe and Central Asia navigate every day. Anthropologists Akhil Gupta and James Ferguson once smartly observed, "The representation of the world as a collection of 'countries,' as in most world maps, sees it as an inherently fragmented space, divided by different colors into diverse national societies, each 'rooted' in its proper place" (Gupta and Ferguson 1992, 6). This clean, "cookie-cutter" view of the world and the shape of human societies within it presents an inaccurate yet tantalizingly digestible view of the nation-states that occupy the former Soviet sphere today. The temptation to adopt this frame has certainly shaped popular understanding of Crimea and Donbas as geopolitical conflicts. After visiting Donets'k, the major urban center of one of the separatist-held regions in eastern Ukraine, the journalist Julia Ioffe noted:

> Maps on television and in newspapers show [Ukraine] conveniently cleaved in half between Ukrainian speakers in the pro-Yulia Tymoshenko [Ukraine's prime minister following the Orange Revolution] west and the Russian speakers in the pro-Yanukovych east. The former love Europe, the latter love Russia. . . . But the truth is more complicated, as it always is. The real split is generational. . . . The younger a citizen of Donets'k, the more likely she is to view herself as Ukrainian [by nationality]. The older she is, the more likely she is to identify as Russian [by ethnicity]. (Ioffe 2014)

As Ioffe observes, there are plenty of distinctions—linguistic, economic, political—that can be used to separate Ukraine's central and western regions from Donbas in the east and Crimea in the south, but within the most seemingly distinct and homogeneous population groups, the very framework through which the concept of *svoi* can even make sense continues, unabated, to evolve.

Clarifying the boundary lines of *svoi* both within and across post-Soviet societies has been one of the largest engines of political discourse in this region since the Soviet era. In Ukraine, sociopolitical battles have been fought over whether Ukrainian deserves the status of a unique language or whether it should be considered a rural dialect of Russian (Bilaniuk 2005), whether urban-dwellers can be considered "authentically" Ukrainian (Peacock 2012), and whether refugees from the war in Donbas could be considered equal citizens (Jones 2014). Economic, ethnic, and linguistic divides in parts of southern Europe have even become so strongly demarcated that some communities have dug up their dead and carried them away to new grave sites to establish, in clear, geographically concrete terms, where *svoi* begins and ends (Verdery 1999).

The lines along which the Ukrainian nation began to divide in early 2014 engaged directly and indirectly with the concept of *svoi* by erasing some of this granularity in Eastern European identities and lifting up certain configurations of *svoi* above others. Crimea, for example, was not a part of Ukraine until 1954, when it was "gifted" to the Ukrainian SSR by Khrushchev in celebration of the three-hundredth anniversary of Pereyaslav, where

Cossack leaders joined forces with Russia's tsarist military forces in their up-rising against the Polish-Lithuanian Commonwealth (Reid 1997). Begin-ning in 1991, Crimea existed as an autonomous region within Ukraine, re-taining its status as the home of a nearly exclusively Russian-speaking population with close historical ties to the Russian Orthodox Church and Russian cultural identity. Since then, as political scientist Eleanor Knott has argued, Crimea has often been viewed by social scholars as nonrepresenta-tive of Ukraine, as an odd-region-out with a particularly pro-Russian politi-cal affinity. These arguments have been based largely on census data that has historically shown the region to be overwhelmingly populated with people who identify as ethnically Russian. However, Knott's own ethnographic re-search among Crimeans around the time of the Russian invasion reveals a much more nuanced system of cultural and political identity, with nearly equal numbers of residents identifying as ethnically Russian and as politi-cally (or nationally) Ukrainian; some also primarily identified as Crimean, an interethnic identity situated somewhere between Russian and Ukrainian (Knott 2015).

Several factors have complicated this softening of ethnic divisions in Crimea. The first is the Russian political rhetoric that frames Crimea as a fundamentally Russian place, drawing lines of distinction not between Rus-sia and Ukraine, as world maps might have us imagine, but between a his-torically imagined "Russian world" and everywhere else. Historian Serhii Plokhy has described this contemporary model of Russian identity as one that "stresses the indivisibility of the Russian nation, closely associated with the Russian language and culture, [and that] poses a fundamental challenge to the Ukrainian nation-building project" (Plokhy 2017, 350). Second, the Russian Federation maintains key military assets in Crimea. The most sig-nificant of these is the Black Sea Fleet in Sevastopol, a vital part of Russian military infrastructure since it was first established by Catherine the Great at the end of the Russo-Turkish War. Today, as then, the fleet provides Rus-sia with precious access to the open seas along its western border—access that requires neither the navigation of Arctic waters nor territorial negotia-tions with Finland, which generally looks unkindly upon Russian naval maneuvers nearby.

Third, as Elizabeth Dunn and Michael Bobick (2014) have noted, con-cern over Russia's proximity to NATO countries has inspired the Kremlin to violate the territorial sovereignty of states in Eastern Europe and Central

Asia in recent years, giving rise to de facto states such as those within the Republic of Georgia and the Republic of Moldova. Since the EuroMaidan revolution began as a protest against the tabling of an association agreement between Ukraine and the EU, it stands to reason that the political victories achieved by the anti-Yanukovych protestors would, from Russia's point of view, be taking Ukraine in the wrong (i.e., pro-NATO) direction. Given this, and given the privilege of hindsight, it was not surprising that Russia began making moves to protect its political and military interests in Crimea when Viktor Yanukovych's ability to regain control over the Ukrainian government seemed all but spent. Remarkably, historian Anna Reid predicted a Russian-Ukrainian conflict over Crimea in the mid-1990s. In her historical analysis of the Ukrainian nation-state, published in 1997, Reid wrote, "Were a civil war to break out in Ukraine, it would most likely begin in Crimea. . . . Were a President Lebed or a President Luzhkov [Russian presidential hopefuls prior to Putin's election to the office in 1999] to successfully re-ignite the se-cessionist movement in Crimea, it would spark a chain reaction into Russian-speaking eastern Ukraine" (Reid 1997, 187). Reid's prognostication was correct on two counts. That "chain reaction into Russian speaking eastern Ukraine" is, in fact, precisely what happened.

In the weeks following the invasion of Crimea, public opposition to the post-Yanukovych government, a government heavily composed of the political and charismatic leaders of the EuroMaidan revolution, rose from a rattle to a boil in the eastern and southern border regions of Ukraine. Protests emerged from Odessa in the south, through Zaporizhzhya, Donets'k and Luhans'k in the Donbas region to the east, and up into Kharkiv in the north. Diffusely branded as "anti-Maidan" movements, this public dissent was fervent and organized—occasionally leading to physical (and sometimes deadly) confrontation with those who supported the revolution and ousted Yanukovych, whose political party enjoyed great popularity in Ukraine's eastern regions (*BBC News* 2014).

These separatist agitations in Ukraine's southern and eastern regions were fueled, in part, by a shared dissatisfaction with quality of life in an independent Ukraine and a shared nostalgia for certain financial securities associated with the Soviet era. Living far away from the actual events of the EuroMaidan revolution in Kyiv, Ukrainians in this region saw recent political actions unfold largely through the lens of Russian-oriented (and often Russian-owned) media, which did not necessarily look favorably on this

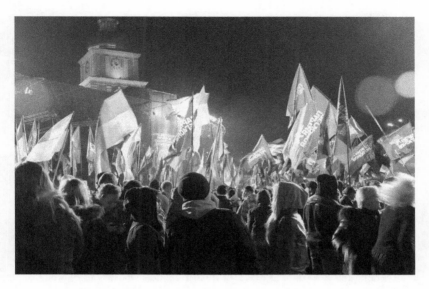

A rally organized in support of the political party of Viktor Yanukovych, the Party of Regions, November 2012. Photo by author.

transition of power. Again, as Ioffe succinctly observed, much was made of the language differences across Ukraine—especially the fact that the Donbas region is predominantly Russian-speaking and largely populated by people claiming Russian ethnicity—in the interest of providing a clean and pithy analysis of these new displays of political unrest. Yet economic and ideological divides are perhaps much more salient than these, as significant disparities between Ukraine's eastern and western regions have grown steadily since Ukraine's independence in 1991 (Skryzhevska, Karácsonyi, and Botsu 2014). Donbas residents, for example, have typically relied more heavily on pension payments and other state services than their western counterparts, a situation that fuels a shared nostalgia for socialist periods, which many often associate with both economic stability and, most importantly, with Russian political control (Skryzhevska, Karácsonyi, and Botsu 2014). As historian Sergei Yekelchyk has observed, "The anti-Maidan struggle was . . . not against Europe per se [as EuroMaidan was, in part, a pro-European movement], but for Ukraine's identity in relation to Russia" (Yekelchyk 2014, 68).

Despite these real concerns plaguing daily life in eastern Ukraine, a study conducted by the independent research organization Kyiv International

Institute of Sociology in 2014 found that only 31 percent of Donbas residents were willing to voice support for some form of secession from Ukraine (Katchanovski 2014). The sentiment was present, but small; something else was needed to push these regions over the edge. Conventional wisdom holds that the alleged indivisibility of the Russian world, as described by Plokhy, was foregrounded in Putin's public discourse specifically to fan these flames in eastern Ukraine (Herszenhorn 2014; Newman 2015; Taylor 2014). For example, in a speech given days after the highly irregular referendum of secession in Crimea, Putin described the reunion of Crimea with the Russian Federation in precisely these terms:

> Everything in Crimea speaks of our shared history and pride. This is the location of ancient Khersones, where Prince Vladimir was baptized. His spiritual feat of adopting Orthodoxy predetermined the overall basis of the culture, civilisation and human values that unite the peoples of Russia, Ukraine and Belarus. The graves of Russian soldiers whose bravery brought Crimea into the Russian empire are also in Crimea. This is also Sevastopol—a legendary city with an outstanding history, a fortress that serves as the birthplace of Russia's Black Sea Fleet. Crimea is Balaklava and Kerch, Malakhov Kurgan and Sapun Ridge. Each one of these places is dear to our hearts, symbolising Russian military glory and outstanding valor. . . . In people's hearts and minds, Crimea has always been an inseparable part of Russia. This firm conviction is based on truth and justice and was passed from generation to generation, over time, under any circumstances, despite all the dramatic changes our country went through during the entire 20th century. (*Washington Post* 2014)

In this way, Putin collapsed the meaning of *svoi* into a singular and timeless Russian identity that could be mobilized for contemporary purposes. In Serhii Plokhy's words, "Russia did not just want the Crimea, it was trying to stop Ukraine's movement toward Europe by manipulating local elites and populations in the east and south of the country" (2017, 341). Putin soon began speaking of large swaths of Ukraine's sovereign territory in similar terms, describing major regions near Kharkiv, Luhans'k, Donets'k, Zaporizhzhya, Kherson, Mykolaiv, and Odessa, as historically Russian (Taylor 2014). Though separatist agitations did not survive long anywhere except the regions of Donets'k and Luhans'k, efforts to rally separatists together did not fail in other regions for lack of effort. Political conflict between Ukrainians who supported the Kyiv government and anti-Maidan activists who pro-moted separatism bled into the streets for weeks and months at a time in eastern Ukraine, and numerous lives were lost as a result (Zinets 2014).

In the promises Putin made in the above speech, and elsewhere, to "pro-tect" Russian-speaking people throughout the region, he chose to refer, for example, to citizens of Ukraine either as Ukrainians or as "natural" Russians, adjusting his framework to meet the needs of his political agenda. It allowed him to bend the operant concept of *svoi* whenever it suited him to do so. This stretch of land reaching from Kharkiv to Odessa, which Putin began describ-ing as historically situated within the Russian *svoi*, was also of strategic impor-tance for Russia's foreign policies and military engagements. The eastern por-tions of the country from Kharkiv to Luhans'k to Donets'k would, if they successfully broke away from the country, provide Russia a significant buffer between its own borders and an increasingly EU-friendly government in Ukraine. The southern regions of Kherson and Zaporizhzhya would pro-vide Russia with a protected land bridge into Crimea, which they now fully controlled, and the regions of Mykolaiv and Odessa would provide a protected land bridge into Transnistria, where Russian troops were still supporting a breakaway region in Moldova. All Putin needed to make the separation of Ukraine along these boundaries seem plausible was a legible configuration of the indivisible Russian *svoi* that unified these lands in a manner distinct from the historical Ukraine. As it turns out, he had one. In mid-April 2014, Putin began referring to all these southern and eastern regions of Ukraine, collec-tively, as *Novorossiia*, the "New Russia" subsumed into the Russian Empire by Catherine the Great in 1774.

Sloviansk

The driving forces behind the crisis in Donbas seem to be apparent. Russian military involvement in these breakaway regions has been exhaustively doc-umented (*New York Times* 2014; Ostrovsky 2015; Schoen 2014). Significant economic, cultural, and political divides placed the EuroMaidan revolution and the sudden regime change in Kyiv in a very different light in different regions of Ukraine (International Republican Institute 2014), and local sup-port for the separatist movement was, to some degree, very real (Babkina 2016). Yet ordinary Ukrainians struggled to make sense of an escalating war in a region that had not seen military conflict since World War II. Most of the Ukrainian military had not been involved in so much as a coordinated exercise since the Afghan war of the 1980s. Many of my own friends in Kyiv and L'viv were devastated as they watched their friends, siblings, and children drafted into the army and sent to fight with little more equipment than what they were able to procure from the local sporting goods store. In response to these collective traumas and uncertainties, a widely held "addiction imaginary" swelled in popular discourse. As a mechanism for assigning blame for the conflict and delegitimizing the separatists' claims to independence, this "addiction imaginary" helped to provide clear, intelligible answers to some of the most difficult questions about the separatist war. More precisely, people who use drugs were cast in the public imagination as the source of the vulnerability that allowed the separatist movement to crystallize in the first place— the loose stitch in the seams that were holding Ukrainian society together.

Sloviansk, a town of about 100,000 located near the northern border of the Donets'k region, is where the violent separatist movement in Donbas got its start. Though this town's involvement in the war lasted a relatively short time, from April 12 to July 5, 2014 (Owczarzak, Karelin, and Phillips 2015), events there managed to wreak havoc on the residents of the town and the infrastructures on which they relied. Trouble began when a faction of armed gunmen stormed the local headquarters of the Security Service of Ukraine. Gunmen were seen wearing the orange and black-striped St. George's ribbon, a World War II symbol that has come to represent contemporary pan-Soviet-cum-Russian nationalism. The office of the Ministry of the Interior in the regional capital of Donets'k was also forcibly seized on the same day (Rachkevych 2014). These events were soon attributed to the organizational leadership of a former Russian intelligence officer named Igor Girkin, a veteran of many other separatist military conflicts within Russia's sphere of influence. In a November 2014 interview with the Russian newspaper *Zavtra*, he stated, "This is my fifth war. There were two in Chechnya, Transnistria [a breakaway region of Moldova], and Bosnia" (Prokhanov 2014). Girkin has a reputation as a fierce and ruthless military operative. He carried out these activities under a well-suited nomme de guerre: "Strelkov" (shooter). Following the establishment of the DNR in the Donets'k region, Girkin was placed at the head of the bourgeoning state's military forces (Sonne and Shishkin 2014).

Outside of the DNR, particularly in those regions of Ukraine situated uncomfortably close to this emergent military conflict, the Kremlin was perceived to be the clear instigator of this violence, having provided the material and human resources necessary to ignite something like a civil war. It was also widely believed that Sloviansk could not have fallen under Girkin's influence as it did without sufficient local collaboration. In this regard, blame was almost universally placed on the illicit drug trade in and around Sloviansk. As recently as 2016, I learned from firsthand reports of many residents (and former residents) of Ukraine's eastern Kharkiv and Donets'k regions that Sloviansk is widely known to be a hub for drug trafficking, providing protected routes for highly desirable substances like heroin and cocaine—drugs that, ironically, few of the individuals living in Sloviansk could ever afford—into Russia and elsewhere. The involvement of corrupt city leadership in these trafficking activities allegedly "primed" them to succumb to Girkin's bribery and promises of power in the new state he set out to create.

This perspective was summed up nicely in a piece of political analysis published in the Ukrainian legal magazine *Konflikty i Zakony* (2014), titled "Answers as to why the separatists chose Sloviansk." The piece outlines three major justifications. First, Sloviansk is located near a major highway connecting Kharkiv, Ukraine's second largest city, with the town of Rostov-on-Don, located roughly sixty kilometers across the Russian border. This bodes well for humanitarian and military supply chains. Second, Sloviansk is quite close to a major railway interchange, which the article describes as an "open path" to administrative centers like Kharkiv, Dnipro, and others. An airfield is also conveniently located in the neighboring town of Kramatorsk, all of which makes Sloviansk a significant infrastructural asset for a fledgling secessionist movement. "Aside from this," the authors note, "Everyone knows that Sloviansk is a military city where drug addiction [*narkomaniia*] has blossomed, especially among the youth." Those who use drugs, the authors argue, are more susceptible to persuasion and more vulnerable to manipulation, are available human resources for any separatist leaders to exploit as they wish. "This is exactly why," the authors explain, "the military checkpoints [in Sloviansk] were manned by such people who were easily manipulable by these means." This is the same logic that cast people who use drugs as socially dangerous spiritual slaves (*raby*) at the Euro-Maidan protests (see chapter 5).

The suggestion that separatist armies were overwhelmingly populated with wanton "addicts" was perhaps one of the most commonly repeated narratives about the war in Donbas. Even Ukrainian military forces often came back from the front with stories of drugged separatists fighting in deadly skirmishes while literally high out of their minds. A military aid group in Kharkiv recounted one such tale, as shared with them by Ukrainian soldiers returning from the front, in its public newsletter. According to these visiting soldiers, local separatist fighters in the DNR and LNR regions were being drugged and "used as cannon fodder" by the predominantly Russian insurgent leaders. "Their checkpoints and barricades are just littered with used syringes," the report reads. "Drugs are brought to them in large quantities from across the Russian border. . . . [The fighters] feel nothing when they are killed" (Hush 2014).

Multiple reports in Ukrainian mass media—most of them citing "anonymous local sources"—also claimed that local residents who use drugs were deliberately, sometimes forcibly, recruited into separatist armies. A popular online newspaper, *TSN*, took to gathering social media reports from individuals living within the DNR to offer evidence of such a claim. "Many able-bodied men refused to obey [separatist] orders and fight against the Ukrainian army," their article reads. "So the soldiers gathered into their ranks those people of low social status: alcoholics, addicts [*narkomany*], and those with criminal records" (*TSN* 2014). Reports also emerged from Sloviansk, specifically, that military recruitment was producing an overabundance of drug use in the DNR's armed forces. One account, first reported by Glavnoe.ua and later reprinted by Ukrainian national news agencies UNIAN and Glavred, not only touched on these issues of substance use but also tied substance use to the pervasive classism that defines the residents of Donbas—especially the young men—as poor, tasteless, and violent. In a word, they are stereotyped as "hooligans." In the report, a local resident is quoted saying, "Do not believe that the residents of Sloviansk are for Russia, for the terrorists. This is not true. Those who walk around in the streets with guns in their hands, they are the local scum: 'addicts' [*narkomany*] and alcoholics. There is not a decent person among them" (Glavnoe.ua 2014).

In all reality, the likelihood that individuals who use drugs constituted a significant portion of the separatist army's biomass is low. As well, the idea that a mass of individuals who must maintain a certain chemical vigilance to control withdrawal symptoms would be uniformly amenable to the regimentation of a separatist military lacks a certain level of plausibility. Political scientist Vera Mironova, who has conducted qualitative research among separatist militias fighting the Ukrainian army in Donbas as well as among insurgent groups fighting ISIS in Iraq, has frequently noted that drugs and war tend to exist in tandem with one another (Mukharji and Mironova 2017). Yet, by her account, substance use problems tend to arise as a result of war, rather than the other way around, as militia leaders often provide stimulants of various kinds to their fighters. "The leaders give their guys the same things, so you can tell who is fighting for which side," she once said "by what kinds of drugs they leave behind" (2016, personal communication). That drugs were present in Sloviansk during the separatist uprising is, therefore, quite possible. The premise that a functioning army could be built with local recruits identified through a preexisting substance use disorder, however, is much less compelling.

How was this vision of a *narkoman* army reconciled with such matters of common sense? The answer, again, is most likely classism. The Donbas region has long carried a reputation as a haven for organized crime. Elsewhere in Ukraine, Donbas residents displaced by war were frequently associated with petty theivery and other social transgressions by those suddenly forced to be their neighbors (Jones 2014). Furthermore, the working class appearance of many young men in Donbas could also be easily misrecognized as outward signs of substance use by those who have been taught to attach stigma to such external signifiers. Sophie Pinkham, a longtime advocate of harm reduction in Eastern Europe, illustrated this point in a recent memoir about her life in Ukraine. "Many of the [Donbas] separatists I saw in pictures and videos looked familiar; these were the same sullen, sunken-eyed young men I'd encountered at harm reduction centers, partial to homemade amphetamines and opiates brewed from Ukrainian poppies. But now they had guns. Now they were heroes" (Pinkham 2016, 207). Yet, where Pinkham seeks to make a broader point about youth, economic insecurity, and political disenfranchisement, many others have seen fit to draw more concrete connections between the stigma of drug use and the outward indicators of poverty. Rather than wrestling with the complex realities that have shaped the economy of daily life in Donbas, one can instead choose to believe that these poor, simple-looking young men had shirked their national heritage for the thrill of a high and the empty promises of violent, foreign instigators. Why shouldn't they be understood as slaves, as zombies, as vacuous *narkomany* available for exploitation by the enemy? How else does one explain why men are laying down their lives to break away from the Ukrainian nation to those who, just months before in Kyiv's center square, laid down their own to protect it?

Serving Sovereignty in a Vigilante State

Ideal configurations of citizenship and citizens' rights in Eastern Europe have long been intimately connected with the social imagination of *svoi*. The protestations of Chernobyl victims who sought care and protection from the state following their radiation injuries is illustrative of this (see chapter 4). When the independent Ukrainian state emerged from the collapse of the Soviet Union, the newly formed government adopted the needs of Chernobyl victims as a banner issue, which, though ill-advised in economic terms, played a key role in Ukraine's reconstitution as an independent nation. By categorically reenfranchising a segment of its population, the independent government was establishing—and projecting globally—the validity of its independent administration. Likewise, the rapid transformation of administrative strategies in contested or de facto states can be interpreted as a form of sovereign "shock therapy"—a method of altering citizens' relationship with the state and reconfiguring the meaning of *svoi* through brute administrative force. For if the sovereign, by definition, is that which has the power to determine who is and is not exceptional, then removing a category of exceptionalism can also be interpreted as an act of state-making. Leaders of the separatist states in Donbas similarly sought to consummate new forms of sovereignty by redrawing the bounds of its citizenry in new ways, redefining who is and who is not *svoi*.

By the summer of 2014, the political metamorphoses of eastern Ukraine's occupied zones were in full swing. The DNR had consolidated into a semi-functioning political organization, and residents of the neighboring Luhans'k region, also under separatist control, had devised the locally-controlled LNR. Flags, seals, and other paraphernalia of Ukraine had long been torn down and replaced with a new iconography representing the new de facto states. Public referenda were held under murky circumstances earlier in the spring, allowing separatist leaders to declare a democratic foundation for independence. The landslide victories declared by separatist leaders—with 89 percent of DNR residents and 96 percent of LNR residents allegedly casting their votes in favor of secession (Gander 2014)—were improbable at best. Igor Plotnitsky, a former reserve officer of the Soviet army and businessman from Luhans'k, seized the presidency of the LNR in November 2014 elections. Aleksander Zakharchenko, a mine electrician from Donets'k, rose to the same position that year in the DNR. Both men took quite naturally to the political theater required of their new public personae. Military man Zakharchenko openly cultivated his image as a noble war hero, while Plotnitsky courted more sensational battles, openly challenging Ukrainian president Petro Poroshenko, who was elected in May 2014 after the fall of the Yanukovych regime, to settle the war by means of a gentlemen's duel (*Moscow Times* 2014).

These men and their administrations adopted a populist approach when posturing their newfound authority before their constituents, doing all that they could to present their meager governments as honorable defenders of the local citizenry. Promises were made (and rumors allowed to circulate) regarding pension increases under the new regime. Many local residents looked optimistically toward the possibility that Russian support would lead to higher payments and a higher quality of life. As all means for collecting state revenue in the occupied zones crumbled in tandem with Kyiv's administrative control, the ability of DNR and LNR leadership to pay higher pensions—or pensions at all—was negligible. Some elderly residents became accustomed to receiving rations of buckwheat and canned meat in lieu of cash payments during the DNR's first year (Weaver 2014). By April 2015, Russia had reluctantly begun floating cash pensions to residents of occupied Donbas while the leaders of these breakaway states maligned the Kyiv government for abandoning its elderly (Åslund 2016). Zakharchenko, for instance, accused Kyiv of "neglecting" its elderly citizens, conveniently omitting that Ukrainian pension distributors—who still distribute pension payments door to door in the form of paper currency—cannot work safely in areas that Ukraine does not control (Donbass International News Agency 2017). Zakharchenko also unilaterally declared all bank debts owed by DNR residents null and void, describing Ukrainian banks as "enemy organizations" that no one should have to pay back (Babkina 2016).

Though the new DNR and LNR governments struggled to make the most basic social services available, they nevertheless identified many other methods for winning over the hearts and minds of Donbas residents and forging a new state in the collective political imagination. The most prevalent of these alternative methods was the concerted, public display of force; within that playbook, the overpolicing of stigmatized social groups was a popular move. Similar to the open displays of violence undertaken by the Internet Party of Ukraine as it raided homes and businesses under the guise of disrupting "drug dealing" operations, the strict public policing of select segments of the population served as a visceral outward manifestation of the sovereign control that DNR and LNR leaders sought to enact. Campaigns to "clean up" local regions of undesirable elements were especially common in the early days of the occupation. In its initial months, DNR leaders established what has been described in media reports as a "pogrom" for local Roma residents (*Donetskaya Pravda* 2014). Reports also emerged of an armed militia storming and looting a gay club in the city of Donets'k (Ukraine News One 2014), and leaders of the LNR went so far as to criminalize homosexuality, threatening sentences of two to five years in labor camps for those convicted (Nemtsova 2014). Police and militia members attacked and intimated local minorities, gays, and various other ne'er-do-wells as part of a low-resource, high-impact strategy for "rebooting" local understandings of the *khoziaistvo* around the new administration and placing sovereign authority squarely in the hands of the new leaders who controlled the police force.

Physically driving alleged *narkomany* out of the DNR and LNR regions was an explicit component of both governments' political agendas (Owczarzak, Karelin, and Phillips 2015). In June 2014, the leader of the LNR militia, Aleksei Mosgovoi, stated that his forces "were bringing order" to the city of Luhans'k. They were preparing, as Mosgovoi explained, to oversee "the wholesale removal of alcoholism and drug addiction from the city and the surrounding villages (Rus: *ochistit' goroda i sela ot poval'nogo alkogolizma i narkomaniia*)." Mosgovoi and his police forces had publicly announced this intent to violently target people who use drugs in this way. "Either you wrap up your 'activities,'" he said, "or we will be coming for you. We have all of your addresses, your family names. . . . You have three days to leave the city. If you do not leave, then only you will be held responsible for what happens next" (Lisichansk.com.ua 2014).

Despite this strong rhetoric from leadership, it was typically separatist fighters of lower rank who carried out many of these threats. In one particularly gruesome example from early 2016, a Russian-born member of the DNR militia (called by the nom de guerre "Olkhon") arrested a man from the town of Kommunar under allegations of drug dealing (it is commonly assumed in Ukraine that anyone who is selling drugs also uses them). The arrestee was bound to a wooden post with duct tape and severely beaten with a long piece of electrical wire, which Olkhon and his partner used as a whipping device. This awful event was captured on shaky, handheld video and posted to an online group of pro-Russian rebels on the social networking site VKontakte (Metro.co.uk 2016). The spoken dialog of this man's abusers is equally chilling. Olkhon can be heard in the video saying, "This is the drug dealer's punishment." "We don't need courts and sentences, this is what we need!" another accomplice cried out. Olkhon continued: "Drug dealers and 'addicts' [*narkomany*], please come here to us, we have a way of dealing with people like you. Come to us and we will cure you all . . . but this fellow will be slaughtered as a dog" (Evans 2016). The arrestee in the video is presumed dead.

Actions such as these made substantial contributions to the perceptions of these separatist governments as formidable (if not legitimate) state entities. The repression of people who use—or allegedly use—drugs was such an effective campaign strategy, in fact, that even Ukrainians living outside the occupied zone could see the logic of it. In 2016 I traveled to Kharkiv with a group of scholars and, while there, met several Ukrainian women who had been organizing a support project for individuals and families displaced by the war. Their work brought them very close to the lived experiences of people fleeing the war. One described that they often met people fleeing their homes the moment they step off the inbound train and onto the platform in Kharkiv. While our group was led on a tour of their agency offices to learn about their work, several members of the staff brought up the topic of people who use drugs near Sloviansk. When asked to elaborate on what they meant, one replied, "Yes, [the seperatists] drove out many 'addicts,' they did do that," one of the women said. "I don't want to say it was a good thing, because I don't want to say that anything having to do with those militias is good. But it was, in a way, some kind of public good." In targeting people who use drugs, then, even these separatist states, which these women denounced as illegitimate and vile, gained a small portion of legitimacy in their eyes. When I asked others about this narrative, many agreed with the women from the aid organization, but didn't take much interest in my line of questioning. More often than not, I was greeted with a polite nod and a shrug. Yes, it's true. They aren't a legitimate state in any way, but at least they are doing this one thing that real states should do.

Sovereignty and Abandonment in Crimea

The selective targeting of people who use drugs was similarly used as a tool for reenacting—or "rebooting"—Russian sovereignty in Crimea. What separated the annexation of Crimea from the separatist war in Donbas, however, was that efforts to remake the Crimean region into a sovereign, non-Ukrainian, administratively Russian state were carried out under the transparent authority of the Kremlin. Where the DNR and LNR relied on select Russian operatives and ragtag "people's militias," Crimea's occupiers were backed by the full political, economic, and military might of a global superpower. Armed with this wealth of financial and human capital, Russian military forces wasted no time in reorienting local mechanisms of sovereign rule away from Ukraine and toward Russia. A new daily reality set in, with different flags dotting public spaces, currency measured in a new denomination, and passports issued in non-European colors.

Among the many administrative adjustments Crimean residents experienced in rapid succession was the realignment of local health-care infrastructure with Russian health-care regulations. Some of these changes have been positive. Reports made to the media outlet *Vox Ukraine* indicate that Crimeans have generally been pleased with various hospital renovations and the availability of new medications free of charge (Talavera 2015). Others have been less warmly received. According to reports from the Kharkiv Human Rights Protection Group, many residents of Crimea who did not gain Russian citizenship after the annexation have since been classified as "foreign nationals," consequently losing their access to health care and other social-welfare services (Coynash 2017; Cumming-Bruce 2017). Yet, regardless of whether individual residents of Crimea experienced these changes as a net gain or a net loss, these measures effectively reset the boundaries of citizenship, reordering the relationship between the sovereign and its citizens and creating a new administratively enforced *svoi*. The Russian Federation was thus able to establish clear sovereign authority over the region by virtue of its ability to create new constellations of inclusion and exclusion.

One of the most sensational changes in health-care policy—which appeared to garner the most international media attention—was the termination of MAT services in Crimea. This decision resulted in numerous patient deaths in the weeks following (Kazatchkine 2014) and has been credited with kick-starting a new HIV epidemic in the region (Roache 2017). I visited several MAT clinics in Crimea over the course of my research. One was the concrete fortress where crosswords were offered in lieu of toilet tissue—one of the most dismal places I saw. Another was the joyful clinic at which I met Masha, Vova, and Dima, where the physicians Ivan and Pavel regaled me with stories of methadone and cucumbers (see chapter 2)—arguably one of the most well-run MAT programs in Ukraine. There was room for improvement, but things were going fairly well for Crimea's eight hundred or so MAT patients. MAT, however, is not offered within the Russian health-care system. The two opioid-agonist medications used for MAT, methadone and buprenorphine, are banned in Russia and cannot even be legally imported ("Rossiiskaya Federatsiya Federal'nyy zakon" 1998). The closure of these clinics, then, served as an administrative correction, allowing Russia a new venue for performing its sovereignty through the enactment of distinctly "Russian" systems of social distinction.

Global health projects, such as Ukraine's internationally funded MAT programs, can also be understood as administrative corrections designed to deliver technologies that ensure health where the allegedly universal "right to health" remains unfulfilled. They become what medical anthropologist João Biehl has called "para-infrastructures": "interstitial domain[s] of political experimentation that become visible in people's case-by-case attempts to 'enter justice'" (Biehl 2013, 422). In this light, internationally funded MAT programs could be seen as an attempt to recast people who use drugs as citizens (albeit citizens of a "counterpublic" that requires special services to manage; see chapter 2) by affording them the "right to health" that this citizenship status should impart. Yet the presence of these para-infrastructures in Eastern Europe signals a particular relationship between the host country and Western discourses of human rights, and subsequently reflects on the limits of sovereignty in the state where those para-infrastructures are placed. As Adriana Petryna and Karolina Follis observe:

> New post-Soviet countries [arrived] late to the game of nation-states, at a moment when the institutional frameworks of states were transforming in the face of globalization. . . . The idea of human rights, celebrated since the end of World War II as the secular "universal moral code" (Morsink 1999), added both hope and volatility to this process. Seeking to expand this code to all humanity following the atrocities of the first half of the twentieth century, the

international human rights movement brought about legal and institutional improvements meant to secure the right of those whose "right to have rights" had been denied. (2015, 403–4)

It has been through this language of human rights that Ukrainian leadership has positioned itself in a profitable relationship with powerful international actors. It has done so, however, by allowing international actors to influence administrative strategies within Ukraine's sovereign borders over which the state would typically have control.

In Crimea, where Russia was actively seeking to undermine any other administrative claims to the region, internationally supported health programs for *narkomany* were, predictably, intolerable to leadership. Russian leaders, too, understand global health institutions as para-infrastructures designed to displace Russian sovereignty over its drug-using population and insert the political logic of human rights, which Russian representatives have been known to criticize (Borger 2016). Indeed, many of the public arguments made by Russian leaders on the topic of MAT in Crimea directly connected these clinics' operation with matters of local sovereignty and citizens' safety. Then-head of the Russian Federation's Drug Control Service, Viktor Ivanov, openly accused local organizations involved with the provision of MAT of "representing the interests of Western pharmaceutical companies" (Bird 2016). In contrast to the "universal moral code" of human rights, which has become the lingua franca of most international diplomacy (Morsink 1999, cited in Petryna and Follis 2015), Russian president Vladimir Putin has sought to wield authority through a single "power vertical," a consolidation of control around a single axis of power: himself (Pertsev 2017). So-called foreign agents, seeking to establish para-infrastructures and "chink the gaps" in the assemblage of administrative strategies engaged by the Russian state as it governs, therefore, constitute ideal targets for state-sponsored censorship under the aegis of that consolidation of power.

The clinic closures happened rather quickly. In mid-April 2014, Ivanov announced his intention to close all MAT clinics in the region in the same speech in which he derided these programs as conduits for Western political interests. This announcement rolled back earlier promises that MAT patients in the region could continue receiving treatment through the end of the 2014 calendar year (International HIV/AIDS Alliance 2014). This delayed termination would still have been less than ideal, but it would have afforded patients and their advocates the time needed to relocate to mainland Ukraine those who wanted to continue treatment and to generate some kind of support plan for those who chose to stay behind or were otherwise forced to do so. Ivanov justified these new plans by citing high levels of drug-related crime on the peninsula. He also argued that the level of drug use in the local population was twice as high as in Russia—a claim that is demonstrably untrue (Heimer and White 2010). Ivanov did not stop, however, at political rhetoric and fuzzy statistical claims. He also described the necessary management of people who use drugs in eugenic terms, saying "the 'rejuvenation' of drug addiction in recent years and the increasing number of female 'addicts' [in Crimea] is causing a rise in the number of births of children with various disabilities, which is a threat to the gene pool." He referred to Crimea's MAT patients as "legalized 'addicts'" and "a serious problem that must be dealt with" (Ivanov 2014).

On May 1, 2014, with eight months remaining in the calendar year and plenty of medications still in stock, all clinics were forced to close their doors. Though Ivanov had stated his intention to see this done only weeks earlier, no date for the planned shutdown was specified. The closures happened, in this sense, without warning and left opioid-dependent patients scrambling. Many scattered in a desperate search for ongoing care. At least sixty left the peninsula for mainland Ukraine, relying on organizations like the Alliance and the All-Ukrainian Network of People Living with HIV to help them through the arduous process of reconnecting with treatment following their sudden relocation (Filippovych 2015). A number of patients moved to Russia, sometimes to rejoin part of their extended family, sometimes with the assistance of Russian authorities who offered to send them to detoxification programs where they could "step down" from their medication (Walker 2015). I have even heard through personal anecdote that some MAT patients traveled as far as Spain to find treatment. How or by what means they ended up there is unclear, but credible sources in Barcelona have insisted they helped no less than four people who had fled Crimea to initiate MAT at a local clinic. Many more MAT patients did not survive the closures. Those who remained in Crimea were left to fend for themselves. Most returned to illicit drugs to manage their methadone withdrawal and self-treat their chronic opioid use disorder. Some chose to end their own lives. Approximately one hundred former MAT patients—more than one in ten—were reported dead by the end of June 2014 (Ingham 2015).

I know through the work of harm reduction organizations in Ukraine that Dima is dead. I learned of his passing while sitting alone at my desk in Seattle, recognizing his face in a public-awareness video that advocated for the plight of Crimean MAT patients. At the end of the video clip, captions revealed which participants in the video had died since its initial filming. If not for his outgoing nature, his eagerness to participate in social projects such as this one, I might never have known what became of him. The whereabouts of Masha and Vova remains a mystery. It is possible that someone at the Alliance knows what happened to them, but I have not been able to obtain this information. Their child, wherever she is, should be preparing to enter the first grade.

Similar to the situation in Donbas, people who use drugs were not the only group singled out by the new sovereign authority. Crimean Tatars, a Muslim minority group, also suffered systematic oppression at the hands of Russian authorities (Human Rights Watch 2017c), and LGBT people are now subject to Russia's strict laws against "homosexual propaganda" and ban on the adoption of children by same-sex couples (Pulitzer Center 2014). Nevertheless, Russian authorities in Crimea continued to pivot their displays of authority around a potent "addiction imaginary" that cast people who use drugs as dangerous agents living outside of, and actively threatening, *svoi*. This strategy was deployed again in late December 2014. Though MAT clinics had been closed for nearly eight months by that time, agents of the Russian Federation's Drug Control Service returned public attention to the abolition of MAT by gathering to incinerate the region's remaining stock of methadone (Ingham 2015). The destruction of these stockpiles was an orchestrated theatrical display, evocative of Yanukovych's anti-drug-trafficking performance in 2010, in which he tried to set fire to illegally purchased samples of marijuana and cocaine in the courtyard of the Ukrainian parliament (see chapter 4). Russian officers, grossly overdressed in Kevlar vests and armed with cumbersomely large automatic weapons, gathered around a furnace to painstakingly place hundreds of bottles of prescription methadone, gathered next to them in a tidy a pile, one by one into a modest fire. Too many of these uniformed men were present: more than were needed to guard the little hill of narcotics and certainly more than were needed to control the furnace and ensure that all the methadone made its way in. The display of authority was heavy-handed. These officers appeared, all too literally, to be waging a war on prescription drugs.

We are able to know what this scene looked like because several photographers were on hand to record it. Photos were published by news outlets worldwide: in English-language media, in Russian-language media, and most important, in the emerging pro-Russian media outlets serving Crimea (Ingham 2015; Kislyakova 2015; Steglenko 2015). The message behind the images was clear: there is a new political order in Crimea. The scene was both a statement about what types of people were acceptable in the new Crimea and a demonstration that the citizenship rights of undesirables could, at anytime, be revoked. Similar to the overpolicing and physical abuse of people alleged to have used drugs in Donbas, the closure of MAT programs and the actual death by flame of the remaining medications was also an attempt to gain the trust and faith of the many by excluding a stigmatized few. To wit, Russian leaders purposefully reestablished state sovereignty in Crimea by excising part of the population framed as dangerous and redefining the bounds of its citizenry.

This, I argue, is what can ultimately be gleaned from the circumstances surrounding Dima's death: a view of the ideological terrain in which those clinic closures took place and the process of state building to which it contributed. As the new sovereign in Russian-occupied Crimea pushed forward new constellations of citizenship, statehood, and *svoi*, distinct from those that came before, so the state's biopolitics, the strategies used to manage the citizenry's individual and collective bodies, and the very concept of citizens' "right to health" were retooled as well. More specifically, MAT patients in Crimea were singled out as a population whose access to essential medicines was restricted, delimiting, in turn, the scope of the "right to health" that would be fulfilled by the state. These individuals were thus forced into a contracted form of citizenship, experiencing disenfranchisement along this single axis of sovereign-subject (or state-citizen) interaction, while ostensibly maintaining all other entitlements afforded by the state to citizens of Crimea.

There Is No Logic to It

In a gray apartment block in Kyiv's Demiivska district, as the sun was setting on a hot July day, I tasted live kvass, richly textured with active yeast colonies, for the very first time. This drink, brewed from stale rinds of old bread, sat fermenting in a large jar on the windowsill. Clumps of organic matter flew to the surface and then plunged to the bottom like tiny jellyfish swimming in a tank. It truly did look "alive."

This chemical operation was overseen by Taras, a bright young doctor who had abandoned his home in separatist-occupied Donets'k to flee with his wife and children to Kyiv. The jar of kvass was a small but precious attempt to reconstruct a feeling of home in a place far away from where home had once been. Taras was the friend of a friend, and through this connection I found myself in his apartment drinking his marvelous kvass and eating a second helping of boiled buckwheat and mushrooms. We had almost arrived too late for dinner, as it took us some time to find the right apartment. Our destination was, in fact, a brand-new apartment for this family: a coveted long-term lease with updated registration papers in one of Kyiv's most convenient neighborhoods. Our meeting was meant to be, in part, a celebration of this monumental achievement, made very difficult by their status as internally displaced persons, or IDPs.

"Work is alright," Taras said as we squeezed around his kitchen table. "Work is alright because I just have to do it. I find patients and make money." Finding everything else they needed to start a new life in Kyiv had been a considerable challenge: registering their children in school, accessing social welfare for the displaced, and even finding a landlord willing to rent to refugees from the east. Taras and his family have fared better than most, but the stigma they bore as former residents of Donbas still weighed heavily on them. IDPs are often stereotyped as criminals or as free riders who refuse to work, and instead plan to live on government support. Taras had even been refused by a previous landlord in Kyiv because, as she said, she "would never rent to *narkomany* like him."

Later, as I walked home with the friend who had brought me to dinner, I questioned him about this story. "I realize that a lot of folks are overly suspicious of people from Donbas," I said, "but what sort of logic would support the conclusion that they're all *narkomany?*"

"There is no logic to it," my friend replied. "It's just, they have no home. They have no job. They have nothing to do. Why shouldn't they be *narkomany?*"

"That doesn't make any sense," I replied.

"No it doesn't," he said. "Like I told you, there is no logic to it. It's just stigma."

This chapter has detailed the many ways in which my friend was correct. The "addiction imaginary" in Ukraine is capable of reflecting so many social fears and anxieties that people who use drugs can be made scapegoats for just about anything. They are the prototypical example of outsiders, agents beyond the limits of *svoi*, perpetual sources of weakness in the social fabric. *Narkomany* fomented the EuroMaidan revolution. *Narkomany* drove the Crimean gene pool to the brink of collapse. *Narkomany* caused the war to happen. *Narkomany* filled the ranks of the separatist armies. And, sometimes, *narkomany* are the only people who can be imagined emerging from Ukraine's domestic war zone. As an index of Ukraine's most formidable threats, even people like Taras are swept up in this panic-stricken refrain.

This chapter has also detailed the many ways in which my friend was wrong. There *is* a kind of logic to the social marginalization of people who use drugs. It is a logic fundamentally rooted in the worldviews that dominate in this part of Eastern Europe. What I am referring to, of course, is the "ethopolitics" (Rose 2007) that measures human worth according to the strength of individual will, producing a moral reckoning and policing of people's inner psychological states.

The institutional empowerment or abandonment of people who use drugs in Donbas and in Crimea served to reify new boundaries of the state, to articulate features in the new relationship between the sovereign and its citizens, and to craft a new nation out of that revised administrative arrangement. And though each of these conflicts has produced tragic results, there is something about Dima's death that I find particularly frightening. Violence in Crimea was not meted out on people who use drugs for the sake of contesting a state government—as separatists in the DNR and LNR contested the authority of the Ukrainian government and attempted to manifest their own. Rather, harm was brought to people with a history of substance use for the sake of *legitimizing* a state government—and a militarily powerful state government at that. The Russian Federation has staked its claims to sovereignty and the scope of its authority on its very ability to deny human rights in this way, and the violence meted out against people who use drugs is nothing less than a demonstration of the state's ability to wield sovereign control over its own citizenry.

Conclusion

Narkomania is an ethnographic portrait of an "addiction imaginary," a culturally contingent theory of socially marginalized people who use drugs that circulates through clinical spaces, legal discourse, public policy, public demonstrations, refugee crisis centers, popular revolution, and theaters of war. Across Ukraine, a localized "addiction imaginary" serves as a template for politically salient forms of distinction. It has given structure to emergent nationalisms. It has facilitated the mapping of social change onto the body politic. It has kick-started the political careers of new states, new sovereignties, and new forms of social order. *Narkomania* also follows this "addiction imaginary" into the mundane spaces of rural clinics and local hospitals, where small but occasionally fruitful efforts are made to extract opioid-dependent people from the hopeless subjectivities this shared imagination would sort them into. This analysis has been framed around several arguments, which I summarize below.

First, "addiction" is a social construct that fills the gap between locally meaningful theories of individual will and our ability to make sense of problematic substance-use behaviors through the lens of those theories. The classic theories of critical medical anthropology suggest that the medicalization of "addiction" might have stripped this condition of its moral connotations, moving substance use disorder out of the realm of individual agency and into the realm of purely biological phenomena (see Rhodes 1996). A quick glance at contemporary media coverage of substance-use issues is sufficient to demonstrate that this potential has not been realized. Public discourse continues to place personal blame on people who use drugs for the injuries or consequences they sustain as a result of their drug use. This is true in the United States, in Ukraine, and elsewhere. *Narkomania* suggests that efforts to medicalize "addiction" have failed to strip away these moral values because the very concept of "addiction" was generated, and is now inseparable, from culturally driven understandings of choice and agency (Valverde 1998). Substance use disorder may be defined by a strict set of clinical criteria, but "addiction" always has been (and likely always will be) modeled around a pathology of the will, constructed to explain why some members of society appear to be making habitual, destructive choices beyond the limits of comprehension and the empathy of most other members of society. The "addiction imaginary" is thus a construct created anew time and time again as different societies chart a clearly defined pathology, which explains how problematic substance use (or any other problematic, compulsive behavior) arises in apparent contradiction to dominant theories of human will.

Second, the production of biomedically defined "Others" within a given society can be equally constitutive of social order as is the creation of ideal, governable subjects. The governability of citizens has long been a central concern of anthropological studies of neoliberalism (Keshavjee 2014). Of note is Stephen Collier's critique of purely theoretical analyses of neoliberalisms, which, he claims, fail to consider what may constitute neoliberalism as a practice and not simply as an abstract ideological arrangement (2011). The analysis presented in *Narkomania* suggests that such practices of neoliberalism can extend beyond the work of city planning, unbundling utilities, and instituting new regimes of commodification (as Collier and others have described) to include the production and enforcement of state policies on health and welfare. Thus, the inequitable distribution of rights—including the use of various administrative tools for the differential management of select portions of society, as seen in the framing of the 2012 version of MoH Order 200 and the cumbersome reporting requirements given to MAT clinics—helps to settle the definitions and the limits of "Othered" social categories and allows state powers to enact their appointed role through the active management of these "Others" for the benefit of the rest of society.

Third, it is possible to establish new forms of sovereignty by enacting new administrative strategies, especially where those strategies are able to redraw the lines of social distinction and enforce new regimes of inclusion and exclusion. Indeed, the ability to create and enforce new categories of social exception was directly and purposefully engaged as a tool of statecraft in Crimea and in Donbas. Those making claims to sovereignty in these contested spaces had unequal access to resources and public platforms at their disposal; however, regardless of whether these proto-states' new "Others" were produced through regulatory force or physical violence, public response both within and beyond their asserted geographic boundaries proves these strategies to be morally and politically compelling to wide swaths of society.

Fourth, both international global health organizations and the local entities they support are easily interpretable as troublesome foreign agents whose activities undermine the sovereignty of their host nations. Michelle Rivkin-Fish (2005), among others, has rightly pointed out the ridiculousness of considering global health, medicine, or even science to be apolitical endeavors. Enacting administrative strategies, establishing infrastructure, and even importing "para-infrastructures" (Biehl 2013) are inherently political projects, as is the choice of a state to accept or resist those projects when foreign actors are seeking to implement them. To this end, global health infrastructures are not only complicit in the reproduction of neoliberal forms of governmentality across global contests; they are also deeply entangled with the domestic struggles among (or between) state powers to produce subjects, produce "Otherness," and enact sovereignty as it is locally conceived. Should state powers decide it is in their interest to contest the authority of that foreign influence the impediment or the outright removal of vital health-care services is an efficient mechanism for achieving this aim.

Lastly, "addiction imaginaries," however they may be constructed, are able to provide symbolically rich and widely legible media to support a state's core sociopolitical projects: the construction of "Otherness," the legal or administrative organization of society around that "Otherness," and the enactment of sovereignty through the violent enforcement of that "Otherness." This is true precisely because the ways in which we formulate our understandings of "addiction" are so closely linked with hegemonic notions of agency, personhood, and the grain of the social fabric. Further, people who use drugs are not alone in their vulnerability to these strategies. In Ukraine, sexual and ethnic minorities are also very much at risk of discrimination and exclusion in nearly all aspects of their lives. In the United States, transgender and non-binary individuals have been similarly targeted by vicious campaigns of "Othering" and exclusion, especially through the sponsoring of so-called bathroom bills that would criminalize the use of a public toilet designated for use by a gender other than one's gender assigned at birth (Kralik 2017). Parallels are readily apparent between "addiction imaginaries" and this "gendered imaginary," which explains away those who do not conform to heteronormative standards of gendered identity as individuals who "refuse" to conform out of some kind of obstinacy or, worse, because they are inexplicable monsters who put the rest of society at risk.

In the final analysis, it becomes clear that these strategies of inclusion and exclusion do not simply tell us something about how "addiction" is viewed in contemporary Ukraine. They also reveal broader patterns of social distinction grounded in sweeping acts of dehumanization and the wholesale rejection of alternative paradigms that seem to contradict broadly accepted understandings of "human nature." By making claims about the liberty with which people are able to use their own minds, the degree to which they are able to think freely, a clear determination is made as to whether such individuals can be considered fully fledged citizens and, subsequently, whether they should be afforded the rights they would be entitled to as such. To achieve full citizenship, people who use drugs and other populations bound by exclusionary "imaginaries" must contend with local ethopolitics (Rose 2007) that produce a sense of stability and order, enjoyed by the majority, by casting these members of "Othered" minorities as living emblems of the emergent social and political threats of the day.

What of Ukraine?

The analysis presented here reveals in stark terms that intense and pervasive social exclusion continues to negatively impact the lives of Ukrainians who use drugs much more than any clinical or individual problem that MAT or other therapeutic interventions can resolve. Despite this, *Narkomania* shows that many patients attempt to alleviate the social exclusion they are subject to in any way they can. Most told me they came to their MAT program because they wanted to live like "normal" people. They grounded their descriptions of this fantastic "normal life" in ordinary details. Normal people make a living wage. Normal people are able to receive good health care. Normal people are able to find work and raise their children. MAT patients tried to manifest these characteristics in their own lives, using MAT as a logistical support for reaching these goals. Overwhelmingly, however, these individuals were unsuccessful in their efforts to position themselves as "normal" people due to the deeply rooted social stigma to which they are constantly subjected.

Recent changes in Ukrainian domestic policy allow for cautious optimism that the quality of life for those most marginalized in Ukraine will improve. Under the presidency of Petro Poroshenko, who took office in June 2014, major efforts to reform the Ukrainian police have been discussed. Under the first deputy interior minister, Eka Zguladze, legislation was proposed that would replace more than 80 percent of the Ukrainian police force in less than five years, thus changing the entire culture of law enforcement in Ukraine ("Ukraine Seeks Foreign Help" n.d.). The first section of law enforcement planned to undergo major changes within the framework of Zguladze's reform efforts is the road police, known for trenchant corruption and exploitation of the public. Training for more than two thousand replacement officers was completed in Kyiv in May 2015 (McLaughlin 2015). So far, these efforts bode well for the future of Ukraine and the safety of its citizens. However, whether or not a hefty turnover in Ukraine's police force will actually come to pass—and whether such a transition will bring an end to police complicity in the illegal drug trade or simply displace those officers controlling the drug trade deeper into the black market—remains to be seen. If the latter occurs, and those currently in control lose their social and professional protections, participation in the informal drug trade, even as a consumer, could become a much more dangerous and more seriously criminal affair.

In late 2016, as the close of what was thought to be the Global Fund's last active grant for the provision of MAT in Ukraine was just weeks away, the government of Ukraine voiced its commitment to fully finance this treatment program with funds from the national budget (UNAIDS 2016). As part of the "willingness to pay" provisions of its grant agreement with the Global Fund, Ukraine was obligated to begin allocating money toward MAT programs in 2016 and to establish dedicated lines of domestic funding in 2017 (Garmaise and Zardiashvili 2016). The government of Ukraine committed USD 31.7million to the national HIV/AIDS control plan, which includes prevention for people who use drugs by means of MAT provision, in 2014. That amount dropped by approximately 50 percent in 2015 and 2016 due largely to the currency crash and financial drain that have accompanied the ongoing war in Donbas. Nevertheless, the Ukrainian government is on track to return to 2014 funding levels in 2017 and 2018 in fulfillment of the agreements made with the Global Fund and PEPFAR to continue providing supplemental funds to pay for essential HIV control programs (U.S. President's Emergency Plan 2017). Historically, actions taken by the Ukrainian MoH—such as the artificially limiting provisions of the 2012 revision of Order 200—have long belied the government's political will to take on the financial and administrative responsibilities of these programs. The post-EuroMaidan government, though subject to seemingly perpetual turmoil of is own, has nevertheless adopted a more cooperative stance with foreign donors of public health assistance.

This commitment to supporting MAT has arisen under the leadership of a new minister of health, Ulana Suprun, a Ukrainian-American physician who relocated from her home state of Michigan to Kyiv to take the position. The administrative changes undertaken by Suprun have been, in a word, sweeping. A new nationwide electronic medical records system was launched in April 2018, which will not only make health records accessible and transferrable in ways never before possible, but will also allow for public health authorities in Ukraine to conduct sentinel surveillance and understand the true nature of disease burdens across the country for the very first time. Many Ukrainians have also gained the ability to choose their own primary care physician, becoming effectively untethered from the polyclinic they had previously been assigned to according to their official residence (Kupfer 2018). The severity of this departure from Soviet approaches to health care cannot be understated.

When I began my research in Ukraine, approximately 8,000 people in Ukraine were receiving MAT. As of February 1, 2018, that number has risen to 10,252 individuals receiving services at 186 different sites. The Global Fund has set the ambitious goal of expanding available services for people who use drugs (including MAT and programs such as syringe access and disposal) to reach 65 percent of the nearly 350,000 individuals in this population in 2017, 70 percent in 2018, and 90 percent by 2020. (U.S. President's Emergency Plan 2018). Access to buprenorphine has also been expanded to primary care clinics, allowing patients to receive these medications from their personal doctor rather than from a narcological dispensary (Morozova et al. 2017).

These are important steps, but many potential obstacles remain. War and internal displacement continues to drain Ukraine's financial resources, and experience of buprenorphine treatment in primary care clinics in the United States shows that increasing availability in this way does not guarantee that more people who need these medications will have access to them— or that doctors will be willing to prescribe them in the first place (Parran et al. 2017). Public statements from Ukrainian officials have reflected a clear understanding that the decision to support or reject essential HIV-control measures like MAT is an ideological one (UNAIDS 2016), and one hopes that the desire to conform to the international expectations held of modern democracies, if not genuine concern for the well-being of its population, will continue to shape the standards of public health and health care for Ukraine's most vulnerable citizens.

What of Russia?

The deadly battles that have swept through eastern Ukraine have spurred new global interest in this region as well as a new wave of political thinking about foreign policies in the post–Cold War era. It is likely, for instance, that Russia's military actions in 2014 made the very concept of Russian meddling in the 2016 U.S. presidential election, which has dominated the U.S. news cycle since, appear plausible to the American public in the first place. Though many violent territorial conflicts have taken place within the confines of Europe in recent years—including wars in Bosnia, Albania, Kosovo, Georgia, and Moldova—much of the Western world nevertheless seemed caught off guard when the territorial sovereignty of Ukraine was challenged by a foreign military. The Russian annexation of Crimea and, to a certain degree, the war in Donbas directly violate the most sacred tenet of the post–World War II European order: that international borders shall not be altered through violence or other means of force. Outrage at these events is fully merited on these grounds alone, and yet, it is difficult to defend the suggestion that this pattern of events is somehow new. The world has borne witness to the military might of multiple nations pressing the boundary lines of European states in one direction or another since the collapse of the Soviet regime. A thoughtful consideration of what drives us to forget these realities again and again is long overdue.

For this reason, ethnographic investigations of post-Soviet modes of sociality, like this one, are desperately needed if our understanding of geopolitical conflict in this region is to improve. Despite (or perhaps because of) our well-developed political understanding of historical tensions between Russia and the European west, Cold War-era paradigms always seem to be coming out of retirement, supporting views of contemporary events that adhere too closely to the social realities of thirty years ago. Today, at a time when human rights has become the dominant language of personhood and now defines appropriate relationships between citizens and states, grounded analyses of medicine, the right to health, and other allegedly apolitical domains of contemporary life must continue to emerge if we are to move beyond obsolete modes of thinking that fail to illuminate anything new about the global political landscape of today.

What this analysis makes abundantly clear is the importance that Russian state authorities currently give to the consolidation of their political control of the former Soviet sphere. This is evidenced not only by the sheer number of soft military engagements and direct military conflicts in which Russia is currently engaged across Eastern Europe and Central Asia, but also the amount of human and financial resources its leadership is willing to sacrifice to territorial conflicts in its "near abroad." Leaked reports indicate that the death toll among Russian ordinary and volunteer fighters in Donbas reached as many as two thousand in the war's first year, alone (Segalov 2015). The human casualties are not limited to those engaged in physical conflict, however. No amount of politicking, diplomacy, or debate can change the fact that Russian authorities deprived over eight hundred people of essential, lifesaving health-care services, passively killing nearly one hundred of those individuals in the process, simply to prove that they could. Russia is actively engaged in the resurrection of its status as a formidable world power, and while many concerns and priorities inform the strategies they employ toward this end, the preservation of life is clearly not one of them.

What of Us?

While still in the process of writing this book, I began working with federal agencies in the United States to combat the ongoing opioid epidemic through the implementation of evidence-based strategies for the prevention and treatment of unintentional opioid overdose. Though I have been working in the fields of harm reduction and substance-use research for the better part of two decades, I still found myself unprepared for the depths and tenacity of the dehumanizing rhetoric used by state and local authorities across the United States to understand and talk about people who use drugs. The idea that living with "addiction" is a willful choice remains alive and well, and that view frequently leads otherwise reasonable people to the conclusion that the greatest U.S. public health crisis since the HIV epidemic of the 1990s is best solved by simply letting people die.

I have become habituated to the constant refrain of voices demanding that people who use drugs be stripped of their most basic civil liberties. Hardly a community meeting or town hall can be held without someone loudly proposing forced hospitalization, involuntary commitment, or compulsory treatment for those living with "addiction." Compulsory treatment does not help. In fact, the science behind compulsory treatment was thoroughly adjudicated by a panel of experts at the National Institute on Drug Abuse (NIDA) in the 1980s. They concluded that compulsory treatment was inefficient, ineffective, and an irresponsible use of public resources (Leukefeld and Tims 1988). NIDA's position on compulsory treatment and involuntary hospitalization has since been reevaluated but has never changed. The evidence continues to tell us what we already know. In the world of clinical research on substance use disorders, this question has long been settled. It is, therefore, incredibly disorienting to be asked to provide expertise on a public health issue, only to be repeatedly contradicted by non-experts who insist that the correct way forward centers around a strategy that has been scientifically disproven for more than thirty years.

What is it, then, that makes us so consistently impervious to evidence-based solutions to our own opioid crisis? What makes us treat people who use drugs with so much ire that we are comfortable stating out loud that their lives are worthless? What is at stake for us when our most deeply held imaginations about substance use in the United States feel challenged? What do our viewpoints about what "addiction" really is accomplish for us, symbolically or ideologically? In the introduction of this book, I asked what social or personal ills in contemporary Ukrainian society MAT seems poised to repair. I asked how the meanings applied to "addiction" and "treatment" in this setting are entangled in broader discourses about power and sovereignty; how these meanings are mobilized in efforts to construct national identity; how the elite subject people who use drugs to selective policing, rights violations, and other delimited forms of citizenship in an effort to exact or consolidate social power. Shouldn't we be asking ourselves these same questions?

A thorough reckoning with our own "addiction imaginaries" is needed if we are to have any hope of quelling the tide of opioid-related deaths across the United States. This is largely because the stereotypes that situate people who use drugs as toxic "Others" are largely self-fulfilling. Marginalization assures that they are systematically stripped of the trappings of ordinary social life. Marginalization keeps them from finding jobs, from finding stable homes, from being at peace with their families, from achieving countless other forms of self-actualization that many of us take for granted. Marginalization is also fueled by an incredible and widespread ignorance about drugs, drug use, and the lived experience of those whose lives have become caught up in these practices. Until more work is done to combat overt discrimination against people who use drugs and to increase their ability to speak openly of their own realities with their own voices, any form of social and clinical support will be palliative, not curative. The change that is needed is social, not clinical. That revolution is still to come.

NOTES

Introduction

1. The names of all informants discussed herein are pseudonyms.

2. The full list of clinical criteria for substance dependence disorder, as listed in the tenth (and current) volume of the International Classification of Diseases is as follows:

1. A strong desire or sense of compulsion to take the substance.
2. Difficulties in controlling substance-taking behavior in terms of onset, termination, or levels of use.
3. A physiological withdrawal state when substance use has ceased or has been reduced, as evidenced by: the characteristic withdrawal syndrome for the substance; or use of the same (or closely related) substance with the intention of relieving or avoiding withdrawal symptoms.
4. Evidence of tolerance, such that increased doses of the psychoactive substance are required in order to achieve effects originally produced by lower doses.
5. Progressive neglect of alternative pleasures or interests because of psychoactive substance use, increased amount of time necessary to obtain or take the substance, or to recover from its effects.

6. Persistent substance use despite clear evidence of overtly harmful consequences, such as harm to the liver through excessive drinking, depressive mood states consequent to periods of heavy substance use, or drug-related impairment of cognitive functioning; *efforts should be made to determine that the user was actually, or could be expected to be, aware of the nature and extent of the harm.* (World Health Organization 2015; emphasis added).

4. *Star Wars* and the State

1. Andriy Klepikov to Raisa Bogatyrova, May 16, 2012.

2. Klepikov to Bogatyrova.

3. Tetyana Alexadrina to the International HIV/AIDS Alliance in Ukraine, May 29, 2012.

4. Dmytro Vorona to the International HIV/AIDS Alliance in Ukraine, June 18, 2012.

5. Inna Emelyanova to Pavel Kupets, July 17, 2012.

6. Inna Emelyanova to the National Council State Service of Ukraine on Combatting HIV-Infection/AIDS and Other Socially Dangerous Diseases, November 5, 2012.

7. Andriy Klepikov to Tetyana Alexandrina, June 21, 2012.

8. Klepikov to Alexandrina.

9. Andriy Klepikov to Viktor Yanukovych, November 29, 2012.

10. Klepikov to Bogatyrova, May 16, 2012; Klepikov to Alexandrina, June 21, 2012.

11. Klepikov to Alexandrina, June 21, 2012.

12. Alexadrina to the International HIV/AIDS Alliance, May 29, 2012.

13. Alexadrina to the International HIV/AIDS Alliance; emphasis added.

14. Oleksandr Tolstanov to the International HIV/AIDS Alliance in Ukraine, September 24, 2012.

15. https://youtu.be/K2JwAHhm6F8.

16. https://youtu.be/H4wVqDf1xks.

17. https://www.youtube.com/watch?v=XcZ1GdDNvfk.

18. https://www.youtube.com/watch?v=0mJjfNoeCSU.

19. https://www.youtube.com/watch?v=VFVFZTrSKh4.

20. Tolstanov to the International HIV/AIDS Alliance, September 24, 2012.

5. The Drugs of Revolution

1. It is not uncommon for adults, especially unemployed adults, to live at home with their parents. Many individuals—including but certainly not limited to those living with a substance use disorder—face a variety of difficulties in keeping their official paperwork up-to-date, meaning that very few of them are properly registered in the apartment where they live. When parents who have official ownership of the apartment pass away, children who are not registered in the apartment do not inherit the prop-

erty. Rather, they lose any legal claim to the residence they may otherwise have had and frequently experience homelessness as a result.

2. This included not only American social scientists but also sociologists and social anthropologists from Sweden, Germany, and Denmark.

3. I am indebted to Jill Owczarzak for this pithy turn of phrase.

4. There are several degrees of disability status in Ukraine. Group I is considered unable to work at all and in need of constant care. Group II does not need constant care, but only special cases are allowed to work. Group III is considered partially disabled and is allowed to work but only on a part-time basis (Phillips 2010, 51).

References

Abdul-Quader, Abu S., Jonathan Feelemyer, Shilpa Modi, Ellen S. Stein, Alya Briceno, Salaam Semaan, Tara Horvath, Gail E. Kennedy, and Don C. Des Jarlais. 2013. "Effectiveness of Structural-Level Needle/Syringe Programs to Reduce HCV and HIV Infection among People Who Inject Drugs: A Systematic Review." *AIDS and Behavior* 17 (9): 2878–92.

Acosta, C. D., A. Dadu, A. Ramsay, and M. Dara. 2014. "Drug-Resistant Tuberculosis in Eastern Europe: Challenges and Ways Forward." *Public Health Action* 4 (Suppl 2): S3–12.

Agamben, Giorgio. 1998. *Homo Sacer: Sovereign Power and Bare Life*. Stanford, CA: Stanford University Press.

Agar, Michael. 1973. *Ripping and Running: A Formal Ethnography of Urban Heroin Addicts*. New York: Academic Press.

American Psychiatric Association. 2013. *Diagnostic and Statistical Manual of Mental Disorders: DSM-5*. Washington, DC: Author.

Åslund, Anders. 2016. "Putin Moves to Direct Rule in the Donbass." *Newsweek*, January 6. http://www.newsweek.com/putin-moves-direct-rule-donbas-412411.

Aspinall, Esther J., Dhanya Nambiar, David J. Goldberg, Matthew Hickman, Amanda Weir, Eva Van Velzen, Norah Palmateer, Joseph S. Doyle, Margaret E. Hellard, and Sharon J. Hutchinson. 2014. "Are Needle and Syringe Programmes Associated with a Reduction in HIV Transmission among People Who Inject Drugs: A Systematic Review and Meta-Analysis." *International Journal of Epidemiology* 43 (1): 235–48. https://doi.org/10.1093/ije/dyt243.

Babenko, L. 1996. "L'épidémie de sida en Ukraine" [The AIDS epidemic in the Ukraine]. *SidAlerte*, no. 54–55 (July): 11.

Babkina, Olena. 2016. "To Be an Inhabitant or a 'Citizen' in the Self-Proclaimed Donetsk People's Republic: A Process of Negotiation of Identities in Discourse and Practices." In *Eighth International Social Science Summer School in Ukraine*. Kharkiv, Ukraine.

Baer, Daniel B. 2014. "USOSCE Statements United States Mission to the OSCE." Vienna, May 12. https://web.archive.org/web/20140512231031/http://osce.usmission.gov/may_8_14_ukraine_roma.html.

Bazylevych, Maryna. 2010. "Prestige Concept Reconsidered: Hybridity of Prestige Concept in Post-Socialist Biomedical Profession." *International Journal of Social Inquiry* 3 (2): 75–99.

BBC News. 2014. "How Did Odessa's Fire Happen?" May 6. http://www.bbc.com/news/world-europe-27275383.

Becker, Howard S. 1953. "Becoming a Marihuana User." *American Journal of Sociology* 59 (3): 235–42.

———. 2015. *Becoming a Marihuana User*. Chicago: University of Chicago Press. http://press.uchicago.edu/ucp/books/book/chicago/B/bo22472239.html.

Belyĭ, S. 2000. "Profilaktika VICH / SPIDa sredi zloupotreblyayushchikh narkotikami i zhenshchin v seks-biznese v gorode Khar'kove" [The prevention of HIV/AIDS among injection drug abusers and women in the sex business in the city of Kharkiv]. *Zhurnal mikrobiologii epidemiologii, i immunobiologii*, no. 4 (August): 105–6.

Benton, Adia. 2015. *HIV Exceptionalism*. Minneapolis: University of Minnesota Press.

Berdychevskaya, Marina. 2004. "Inektsiya zhizni" [Injection of life]. *Korrespondent*, March 20.

Bereza, Anastasiya. 2013. "Volonter Liza: Chelovek neogranichennykh vozmozhnostey" [Volunteer Liza: someone with unlimited abilities]. *Ukrainska Pravda*, December 16. http://life.pravda.com.ua/person/2013/12/16/145837/.

Biehl, João. 2013. "The Judicialization of Biopolitics: Claiming the Right to Pharmaceuticals in Brazilian Courts." *American Ethnologist* 40 (3): 419–36.

Bilaniuk, Laada. 2005. *Contested Tongues: Language Politics and Cultural Correction in Ukraine*. Ithaca, NY: Cornell University Press.

Bird, Michael. 2016. "Crimea: Where Russia's War on Drugs Has Deadly Consequences." The Black Sea: Diving Deep into Stories. February 25. https://theblacksea.eu/index.php?idT=88&idC=88&idRec=1226&recType=story.

Bluthenthal, Ricky N., Greg Ridgeway, Terry Schell, Rachel Anderson, Neil M. Flynn, and Alex H. Kral. 2007. "Examination of the Association between Syringe Exchange Program (SEP) Dispensation Policy and SEP Client-Level Syringe Coverage among Injection Drug Users." *Addiction* 102 (4): 638–46.

Bojko, Martha J., Sergii Dvoriak, and Frederick L. Altice. 2013. "At the Crossroads: HIV Prevention and Treatment for People Who Inject Drugs in Ukraine." *Addiction* 108 (10): 1697–99.

Bojko, Martha J., Alyona Mazhnaya, Iuliia Makarenko, Ruthanne Marcus, Sergii Dvoriak, Zahedul Islam, and Frederick L. Altice. 2015. "'Bureaucracy & Beliefs': Assessing the Barriers to Accessing Opioid Substitution Therapy by People Who Inject Drugs in Ukraine." *Drugs: Education, Prevention, and Policy*, March, 1–8.

Bonn, Dorothy. 2004. "Ukraine's HIV/AIDS Programme Rescued." *Lancet Infectious Diseases* 4 (4): 192.

Booth, Robert E., Jane Kennedy, Tom Brewster, and Oleg Semerik. 2003. "Drug Injectors and Dealers in Odessa, Ukraine." *Journal of Psychoactive Drugs* 35 (4): 419–26.

Borger, Julian. "Russia Denied Membership of UN Human Rights Council." *Guardian*, October 28, 2016. https://www.theguardian.com/world/2016/oct/28/russia-denied-membership-of-un-human-rights-council. Accessed October 26, 2018.

Bourgois, Philippe. 2000. "Disciplining Addictions: The Bio-Politics of Methadone and Heroin in the United States." *Culture, Medicine and Psychiatry* 24 (2): 165–95.

———. 2003. *In Search of Respect: Selling Crack in El Barrio*. Cambridge: Cambridge University Press.

Bourgois, Philippe, and Jeffrey Schonberg. 2009. *Righteous Dopefiend*. Berkeley: University of California Press.

Brave Heart, Maria Yellow Horse. 2003. "The Historical Trauma Response among Natives and Its Relationship with Substance Abuse: A Lakota Illustration." *Journal of Psychoactive Drugs* 35 (1): 7–13.

Butler, Judith. 2007. "From Bodies That Matter." In *Beyond the Body Proper: Reading the Anthropology of Material Life*, edited by Margaret Lock and Judith Farquhar, 164–75. Durham, NC: Duke University Press.

Caldwell, Melissa L. 2004. *Not by Bread Alone: Social Support in the New Russia*. Berkeley: University of California Press.

Callon, Michel. 1986. "Some Elements of the Sociology of Translation: Domestication of the Scallops and the Fishermen of St Brieuc Bay." In *Power, Action, and Belief: A New Sociology of Knowledge?* edited by John Law, 32:196–233. Sociological Review Monographs. Boston: Routledge and Kegan Paul.

Campbell, Nancy D. 2007. *Discovering Addiction: The Science and Politics of Substance Abuse Research*. Ann Arbor: University of Michigan Press.

Carr, E. Summerson. 2010. *Scripting Addiction: The Politics of Therapeutic Talk and American Sobriety*. Princeton, NJ: Princeton University Press.

Carroll, Jennifer J. 2011. "A Woman among Addicts: The Production and Management of Identities in a Ukrainian Harm Reduction Program." *Anthropology of East Europe Review* 29 (1): 23–34.

———. 2013. "Barriers to Treatment Adherence in Ukrainian Tuberculosis Control Programs." Research brief. IREX. https://www.irex.org/sites/default/files/Carroll%20Research%20Brief.pdf.

———. 2016a. "Da vodish normalen zhivot: Komentary vrkhu revolyutsiyata, kolektivnostta, i sotsialnata distinktsiya v Ukrayna" [To live a normal life: notes on revolution, collectivity, and social distinction in Ukraine]. *Kritija y khumanism* 44 (1–2): 69–88.

———. 2016b. "Why Does Healthcare for People Who Use Drugs in Ukraine Continue to Fail?" October 2016. https://krytyka.com/en/ukraines-public-health-challenge/articles/why-does-healthcare-people-who-use-drugs-ukraine-continue.

Carroll, Jennifer J., Brandon D. L. Marshall, Josiah D. Rich, and Traci C. Green. 2017. "Exposure to Fentanyl-Contaminated Heroin and Overdose Risk among Illicit Opioid Users in Rhode Island: A Mixed Methods Study." *International Journal of Drug Policy* 46: 136–45.

Chapman, Rachel R., and Jean R. Berggren. 2005. "Radical Contextualization: Contributions to an Anthropology of Racial/Ethnic Health Disparities." *Health* 9 (2): 145–67.

Chernichkin, Kostyantyn. 2014. "Ukraine's Prosecutor General Classifies Self-Declared Donetsk and Luhansk Republics as Terrorist Organizations." May 16. http://www .kyivpost.com/article/content/ukraine-politics/ukraines-prosecutor-general-classifies -self-declared-donetsk-and-luhansk-republics-as-terrorist-organizations-348212 .html.

Chilingaryan, L. I. 1999. "Teoria I. P. Pavlova o vyschey nervnoy deyatel'nosti: vekhi i tendentsii razbitya" [Pavlov's theory of higher order nervous activity: milestones and trends of development]. *Zhurnal vyschey nervnoy deyatel'nosti* 49 (6): 898–908.

Chybisov, Andriy. 2016. "LGBTQ Discussions in Ukraine: Now Is the Right Time." *Krytika*, October. https://krytyka.com/en/ukraines-public-health-challenge/articles/lgbtq -discussions-ukraine-now-right-time.

Ciccarone, Daniel. 2009. "Heroin in Brown, Black and White: Structural Factors and Medical Consequences in the US Heroin Market." *International Journal of Drug Policy* 20 (3): 277–82.

Cohen, Jon. 2010. "Law Enforcement and Drug Treatment: A Culture Clash." *Science* 329 (5988): 169.

Collier, Stephen J. 2011. *Post-Soviet Social: Neoliberalism, Social Modernity, Biopolitics.* Princeton, NJ: Princeton University Press.

Collins, Chris, and Chris Beyrer. 2013. "Country Ownership and the Turning Point for HIV/AIDS." *Lancet Global Health* 1 (6): e319–20.

Cornish, Rosie, John Macleod, John Strang, Peter Vickerman, and Matt Hickman. 2010. "Risk of Death during and after Opiate Substitution Treatment in Primary Care: Prospective Observational Study in UK General Practice Research Database." *BMJ: British Medical Journal* 341.

Coynash, Halya. 2017. "Ukrainian Citizens Turned into 'Foreign Nationals' in Russian-Occupied Crimea." Kharkiv Human Rights Protection Group, October 31, 2017. http://khpg.org/en/index.php?id=1509032894.

Crane, Johanna Tayloe. 2013. *Scrambling for Africa: AIDS, Expertise, and the Rise of American Global Health Science.* Ithaca, NY: Cornell University Press.

Cumming-Bruce, Nick. 2017. "Russia Committed 'Grave' Rights Abuses in Crimea, U.N. Says." *New York Times*, September 25. https://www.nytimes.com/2017/09/25/world /europe/russia-crimea-un.html.

Dai, Bingham. 1937. *Opium Addiction in Chicago.* Montclair, NJ: Patterson Smith.

Davoli, Marina, Anna M. Bargagli, Carlo A. Perucci, Patrizia Schifano, Valeria Belleudi, Matthew Hickman, Giuseppe Salamina, et al. 2007. "Risk of Fatal Overdose during and after Specialist Drug Treatment: The VEdeTTE Study, a National Multi-Site Prospective Cohort Study." *Addiction* 102 (12): 1954–59.

Degenhardt, Louisa, Deborah Randall, Wayne Hall, Matthew Law, Tony Butler, and Lucy Burns. 2009. "Mortality among Clients of a State-Wide Opioid Pharmacotherapy Program over 20 Years: Risk Factors and Lives Saved." *Drug and Alcohol Dependence* 105 (1–2): 9–15.

De Rond, Mark. 2017. *Doctors at War: Life and Death in a Field Hospital.* The Culture and Politics of Health Care Work. Ithaca, NY: Cornell University Press.

Dole, V. P., M. E. Nyswander, and M. J. Kreek. 1966. "Narcotic Blockade: A Medical Technique for Stopping Heroin Use by Addicts." *Transactions of the Association of American Physicians* 79: 122–36.

Donbass International News Agency. 2017. "Zakharchenko: Kiev Owes Donbass $1.1 Bln in Pensions." March 23. https://dninews.com/article/zakharchenko-kiev-owes-donbass-11-bln-pensions.

Donetskaya Pravda. 2014. "Separatisty obyasnili pogromy Romov v Slavyanske." [Separatists discuss Roma pogroms in Slovyansk]. *Donetskaya Pravda,* April 20. http://novosti.dn.ua/news/206145-separatysty-obyasnyly-pogromy-romov-v-slavyanske.

Driscoll, Jesse. 2015. *Warlords and Coalition Politics in Post-Soviet States.* New York: Cambridge University Press.

Du Bois, W. E. Burghardt. 1998. *Black Reconstruction in America, 1860–1880.* New York: Free Press.

Dunn, Elizabeth C. 2004. *Privatizing Poland.* Ithaca, NY: Cornell University Press.

———. 2008. "Standards and Person-Making in East Central Europe." In *Global Assemblages,* edited by Aihwa Ong and Stephen J. Collier, 173–93. Malden, MA: Blackwell.

Dunn, Elizabeth C., and Michael S. Bobick. 2014. "The Empire Strikes Back: War without War and Occupation without Occupation in the Russian Sphere of Influence." *American Ethnologist* 41 (3): 405–13.

Durkheim, Emile. 1979. *Suicide.* New York: Free Press.

Durning, Dan. 2014. "Celebrating Ukraine's Orange Revolution: Photos of Inauguration Day, Kiev, January 23, 2005." *Eclectic (At Best)* (blog), January 22. http://www.eclecticatbest.com/2014/01/celebrating-ukraines-orange-revolution.html.

Evans, Sophie. 2016. "'Drug Dealer' Beaten with Electrical Cables and 'Tortured' by pro-Russian Rebels." *Mirror,* February 16. http://www.mirror.co.uk/news/world-news/drug-dealer-beaten-electrical-cables-7378585.

Fehérváry, Krisztina. 2002. "American Kitchens, Luxury Bathrooms, and the Search for a 'Normal' Life in Postsocialist Hungary." *Ethnos* 67 (3): 369–400.

Field, John M., Peter J. Kudenchuk, Robert O'Connor, and Terry VandenHoek. 2012. *The Textbook of Emergency Cardiovascular Care and CPR.* Lippincott Williams and Wilkins.

Field, Mark G. 1953. "Some Problems of Soviet Medical Practice: A Sociological Approach." *New England Journal of Medicine* 248 (22): 919–26.

———. 1967. *Soviet Socialized Medicine: An Introduction.* New York: Free Press.

Filippovych, Sergii. 2015. "Impact of Armed Conflicts and Warfare on Opioid Substitution Treatment in Ukraine: Responding to Emergency Needs." *International Journal of Drug Policy* 26 (1): 3–5.

Foley, P. J. 1998. "Is the World Paying Enough Attention to the AIDS Epidemic in Ukraine and Other Newly Independent States?" *Social Marketing Quarterly* 4 (3): 7–12.

Foucault, Michel. 1977. *Discipline and Punish: The Birth of the Prison.* Vintage Books.

———. 1982. "The Subject and Power." *Critical Inquiry* 8 (4): 777–95.

Fournier, Anna. 2012. *Forging Rights in a New Democracy: Ukrainian Students between Freedom and Justice*. University of Pennsylvania Press.

Gander, Kashmira. 2014. "Ukraine Crisis: Russia Backs Results of Sunday's Referendums In." *The Independent*, May 12. http://www.independent.co.uk/news/world/europe /ukraine-crisis-russia-backs-results-of-sundays-referendums-in-donetsk-and -luhansk-9354683.html.

Garcia, Angela. 2010. *The Pastoral Clinic: Addiction and Dispossession along the Rio Grande*. Berkeley: University of California Press.

Garmaise, David, and Tina Zardiashvili. 2016. "Global Fund Reminds Ukraine of Its Commitment to Take Over the Funding of MST | Aidspan." September 4. http://www .aidspan.org/gfo_article/global-fund-reminds-ukraine-its-commitment-take-over -funding-mst.

Garrett, Laurie. 2007. "The Challenge of Global Health." *Foreign Affairs*, January 1. https://www.foreignaffairs.com/articles/2007-01-01/challenge-global-health.

Garriott, William Campbell. 2011. *Policing Methamphetamine: Narcopolitics in Rural America*. New York: New York University Press.

Garriott, William, and Eugene Raikhel. 2015. "Addiction in the Making." *Annual Review of Anthropology* 44 (1): 477–91.

Gessen, Masha. 2017. *The Future Is History: How Totalitarianism Reclaimed Russia*. New York: Riverhead Books.

Glavnoe.ua. 2014. "Zhitel' Slavyanska: za poselednie dva dna gorod pokinuli minimum 400 avtomobiley" [Resident of Slovyansk: more than 400 cars have left in the last 2 days]." Glavnoe.Ua. May 7. http://glavnoe.ua/news/n175786.

The Global Fund to Fight AIDS, Tuberculosis, and Malaria (Global Fund). 2010. "Ukraine: Country Grant Portfolio." https://www.theglobalfund.org/en/portfolio /country/grant/?k=7d5c0bfd-a95b-43d3-bc73-cc862c7b0af5&grant=UKR-102-G04 -H-00.

The Global Fund to Fight AIDS, Tuberculosis, and Malaria (Global Fund). 2012. "Monitoring and Evaluation." http://www.theglobalfund.org/en/activities/monitoringevaluation/.

The Global Fund to Fight AIDS, Tuberculosis, and Malaria (Global Fund). 2016a. "Global Fund Overview." http://www.theglobalfund.org/en/overview/.

The Global Fund to Fight AIDS, Tuberculosis, and Malaria (Global Fund). 2016b. "Government Donors." http://www.theglobalfund.org/en/government/.

Goffman, Erving. 1963. *Stigma: Notes on the Management of Spoiled Identity*. New York: Simon and Schuster.

Golovanevskaya, Maria, Leonid Vlasenko, and Roxanne Saucier. 2012. "In Control? Ukrainian Opiate Substitution Treatment Patients Strive for a Voice in Their Treatment." *Substance Use and Misuse* 47 (5): 511–21.

Gorskaya, Dariya. 2013. "Liza Shaposhnik: 'Tol'ko na maydane vervye pochubstvovala sebya polnotsennoy, zhelannoy y lyubimoy'" [Liza Shaposhnik: 'Only at Maidan did I feel full, desired, and loved for the first time']. *Fakty.Ua*, December 19. http:// fakty.ua/173943-liza-shaposhnik-tolko-na-majdane-vpervye-pochuvstvovala-sebya -polnocennoj-zhelannoj-i-lyubimoj.

———. 2015. "Liza Shaposhnik: 'Mne seychas ne do razborok: ya dolzhna vynosit' i rodit' dvoynyu'" [Liza Shaposhnik: 'I don't have time for fighting: I should get pregnant and

have twins']. *Fakty.Ua*. http://fakty.ua/207257-liza-shaposhnik-mne-sejchas-ne-do
-razborok-ya-dolzhna-vynosit-i-rodit-dvojnyu.

Grissinger, Matthew. 2011. "Keeping Patients Safe from Methadone Overdoses." *Pharmacy and Therapeutics* 36 (8): 462–66.

Grund, Jean-Paul C., Alisher B. Latypov, and Magdalena Harris. 2013. "Breaking Worse: The Emergence of Krokodil and Excessive Injuries among People Who Inject Drugs in Eurasia." *International Journal of Drug Policy* 24 (4): 265–74.

Gupta, Akhil, and James Ferguson. 1992. "Beyond 'Culture': Space, Identity, and the Politics of Difference." *Cultural Anthropology* 7 (1): 6–23.

Hamers, F. F., V. Batter, A. M. Downs, J. Alix, F. Cazein, and J. B. Brunet. 1997. "The HIV Epidemic Associated with Injecting Drug Use in Europe: Geographic and Time Trends." *AIDS* 11 (11): 1365–74.

Harding, Luke. 2010. "Ukraine Parliamentary Vote on Black Sea Fleet Erupts into Fistfight." *The Guardian*, April 27. https://www.theguardian.com/world/2010/apr/27/ukraine-parliament-fight-eggs.

Heimer, Robert, and Edward White. 2010. "Estimation of the Number of Injection Drug Users in St. Petersburg, Russia." *Drug and Alcohol Dependence* 109 (1–3): 79–83.

Herszenhorn, David M. 2014. "What Is Putin's 'New Russia'?" *New York Times*, April 18. https://www.nytimes.com/2014/04/19/world/europe/what-is-putins-new-russia.html.

Hrycak, Alexandra. 2006. "Foundation Feminism and the Articulation of Hybrid Feminisms in Post-Socialist Ukraine." *East European Politics and Societies* 20 (1): 69–100.

——. 2007. "From Global to Local Feminisms: Transnationalism, Foreign Aid and the Women's Movement in Ukraine." In *Sustainable Feminisms*, 11:75–93. Advances in Gender Research. Bingley: Emerald Group.

Human Rights Watch. 2006. "Rhetoric and Risk: Human Rights Abuses Impeding Ukraine's Fight against HIV/AIDS." http://hrw.org/reports/2006/ukraine0306/ukraine0306web.pdf.

——. 2011. "Human Rights Watch: Ukraine—Stop Targeting Harm Reduction Services." Harm Reduction International. February 10. https://www.hri.global/contents/862.

——. 2017a. "Ukraine: Urgent Need for Accountability." January 12. https://www.hrw.org/news/2017/01/12/ukraine-urgent-need-accountability.

——. 2017b. "Human Rights Watch Country Profiles: Sexual Orientation and Gender Identity." June 23. https://www.hrw.org/news/2017/06/23/human-rights-watch-country-profiles-sexual-orientation-and-gender-identity.

——. 2017c. "Online and on All Fronts | Russia's Assault on Freedom of Expression." July 18. https://www.hrw.org/report/2017/07/18/online-and-all-fronts/russias-assault-freedom-expression.

Humphrey, Caroline. 2002. *The Unmaking of Soviet Life: Everyday Economies After Socialism*. Ithaca, NY: Cornell University Press.

Hush, Yuliya. 2014. "Kharkiv'ky muzikanty zihraly dlya poranenykh viys'kovykh" [Kharkiv musicians played for wounded soldiers]. *Spravzhnya varta*, August 14. http://varta.kharkov.ua/news/city/1102346.html.

Hutchinson, The Honorable Asa. 2002. "Narco-Terror: The International Connection between Drugs and Terror." The Heritage Foundation, June 20. https://www.heritage

.org/homeland-security/report/narco-terror-the-international-connection-between-drugs-and-terror.

Hyde, L. 1999. "HIV and Drug Users in Ukraine: Building Confidence to Reduce HIV Risk." *Impact on HIV* 1 (2): 3–7.

Ingham, Richard. 2015. "AIDS Crisis Brewing in Crimea and East Ukraine Says UN." January 20. http://news.yahoo.com/aids-crisis-brewing-crimea-east-ukraine-says-un-002934023.html.

Inspired.com.ua. 2014. "#Yevromaydan: istoriyi spravzhnikh heroyiv." [EuroMaidan: a history of true heroes]. http://inspired.com.ua/people/euromaidan-heroes/.

Interfax-Ukraine. 2010. "Justice Ministry Registers Internet Party of Ukraine." KyivPost. April 6. https://www.kyivpost.com/article/content/ukraine-politics/justice-ministry-registers-internet-party-of-ukrai-63274.html.

International HIV/AIDS Alliance in Ukraine. 2010. "Police Exert More Pressure on Medics and Patients." http://www.aidsalliance.org.ua/ru/news/pdf/03062010/PRESS_RELEASE_ENG.doc.

———. 2014. "Nakazano vyzhyty: poryatunok patsiientiv-bizhentsiv z Krymu ta Donbasu." [Punished for living: saving patient-refugees from Crimea and Donbas]. http://www.aidsalliance.org.ua/ru/news/pdf/06-2014/19.06.2014/Release_19%2006%202014_UNIAN_OST.docx.

International Republican Institute. 2014. "Public Opinion Survey Residents of Ukraine: March 14–26." International Republican Institute, funded by USAID. http://www.iri.org/sites/default/files/2014 April 5 IRI Public Opinion Survey of Ukraine, March 14-26, 2014.pdf.

The Internet Party of Ukraine. 2009a. "Charter." http://ipu.com.ua/page/Ustav/.

The Internet Party of Ukraine. 2009b. "Program." http://www.ipu.com.ua/page/Programma/.

"Interview with the Global Fund to Fight AIDS, Tuberculosis and Malaria." 2005. IRIN, December 29. http://www.irinnews.org/fr/node/198483.

Ioffe, Julia. 2014. "Eastern Ukraine Is Still Fighting Its Past." *New Republic*, March 6. https://newrepublic.com/article/116897/eastern-ukraines-history-under-stalin-holding-it-back.

Ivanov, Viktor. 2014. "Vystuplenie predsedatelya Gosudarstvennogo antinarkoticheskogo komiteta, direktora FSKN Rossii V. P. Ivanova na Vyezdnom soveshchanii predsedatelya GAK 'O perfoocherednykh sadachakh po realizatsii Strategii gosudarstvennoy antinarkoticheskoy politiki v subyektakh Rossiyskoy Federatsii Krymskogo federal'nogo okruga' (g. Simferopol' 2 Apr 2014)." [Speech of the out-going head of the state anti-drug committee, director of the National Drug Control service, V. P. Ivanov, 'Performance measures for the implementation of the state anti-drug political strategy regarding the Crimean Federal District of the Russian Federation' (Simferopol, April 2, 2014)]. Simferopol. http://fskn.gov.ru/includes/periodics/speeches_fskn/2014/0402/104829810/detail.shtml.

Jones, Deborah. 2014. "'They Treated Us Like We Were from Donbass': Displacement and 'Self-Reliance' in Odessa, Autumn 2014." *Perspectives on Europe* 44 (2): 9–14.

Joseph, Herman, and Phil Appel. 1993. "Historical Perspectives and Public Health Issues." State Methadone Treatment Guidelines: Treatment Improvement Protocol

(TIP) Series #1. Rockville, MD: Substance Abuse and Mental Health Services Administration. http://www.ctcertboard.org/files/TIP1.pdf.

Katchanovski, Ivan. 2014. "What Do Citizens of Ukraine Actually Think about Secession?" *Washington Post*, July 20. https://www.washingtonpost.com/news/monkey-cage/wp/2014/07/20/what-do-citizens-of-ukraine-actually-think-about-secession/.

Kazatchkine, M. 2014. "Russia's Ban on Methadone for Drug Users in Crimea Will Worsen the HIV/AIDS Epidemic and Risk Public Health." *BMJ: British Medical Journal* 348 (May 8): g3118.

Keshavjee, Salmaan. 2014. *Blind Spot: How Neoliberalism Infiltrated Global Health*. Berkeley: University of California Press.

Kislyakova, Anastasia. 2015. "Perekhod na myagkuyu silu" [The switch to soft power]. Lenta.Ru., April 24. https://lenta.ru/articles/2015/04/22/drugsbrics/.

Kleinman, Arthur. 1988. *The Illness Narratives: Suffering, Healing, and the Human Condition*. New York: Basic Books.

Knott, Eleanor. 2015. "Generating Data: Studying Identity Politics from a Bottom-Up Approach in Crimea and Moldova." *East European Politics and Societies* 29 (2): 467–86.

Kobyshcha, Iu. 1999. "Determinanty rasprostraneniya VICH sredi narkomanov v Ukraine." [The determinants of the spread of HIV among injection drug addicts in Ukraine]. *Zhurnal mikrobiologii, epidemiologii i immunobiologii*, no. 1 (February): 34–36.

Koch, Erin. 2013. *Free Market Tuberculosis: Managing Epidemics in Post-Soviet Georgia*. Nashville, TN: Vanderbilt University Press.

Konflikty i Zakony. 2014. "Otvet, pochemu separatisty vybrali Slavyansk" [An answer to the question of why separatists took Slovyansk]. *Konflikty i Zakony*, April 17. http://k-z.com.ua/ukrayna/30336-otvet-pochemu-separatisty-vybrali-slavyansk.

Kosten, Thomas R., and Tony P. George. 2002. "The Neurobiology of Opioid Dependence: Implications for Treatment." *Science and Practice Perspectives* 1 (1): 13–20.

Kralik, Joellen. 2017. "'Bathroom Bill' Legislative Tracking." National Conference of State Legislatures, July 28. http://www.ncsl.org/research/education/-bathroom-bill-legislative-tracking635951130.aspx.

Kupfer, Mathew. 2018. "Medical Reform Proves to Be Divisive, Complicated." *KyivPost*, May 4. https://www.kyivpost.com/business/medical-reform-proves-divisive-complicated.html.

Kuzio, Taras. 2006. "Everyday Ukrainians and the Orange Revolution." In *Revolution in Orange: The Origins of Ukraine's Democratic Breakthrough*, edited by Ånders Aslund and Michael McFaul, 45–68. Washington, DC: Carnegie Endowment for International Peace.

Laessig, Gavon. 2011. "Seriously, Don't Use Krokodil." BuzzFeed. http://www.buzzfeed.com/gavon/seriously-dont-use-krokodil.

Latypov, Alisher B. 2011. "The Soviet Doctor and the Treatment of Drug Addiction: 'A Difficult and Most Ungracious Task.'" *Harm Reduction Journal* 8(32).

Ledeneva, Alena. 2006. *How Russia Really Works: The Informal Practices That Shaped Post-Soviet Politics and Business*. Ithaca, NY: Cornell University Press.

Leukefeld, C. G., and F. M. Tims. 1988. "Compulsory Treatment: A Review of Findings." *NIDA Research Monograph* 86: 236–51.

Lindesmith, Alfred Ray. 1947. *Opiate Addiction*. Bloomington, IN: Principia Press.

———. 1968. *Addiction and Opiates*. Chicago: Aldine.

Lisichansk.com.ua. 2014. "V Lisichanske opolchentsy dali tri dnya narkodileram, chtoby uyti iz goroda" [Militia in Lisichansk give drug dealers 3 days to leave town]. July 4. http://lisichansk.com.ua/2014/06/29949.

"Liza Shaposhnik: The Main Drop in the Ocean of EuroMaidan." n.d. Facebook. Accessed October 27, 2014. https://www.facebook.com/pages/Ліза-Шапошнік -головна-крапля-в-океані-Євромайдану/258577444294644?sk=info.

Lovell, Anne M. 2013. "Elusive Travelers: Russian Narcology, Transnational Toxicomanias, and the Great French Ecological Experiment." In *Addiction Trajectories*, edited by Eugene Raikhel and William Garriott, 126–59. Durham, NC: Duke University Press.

MacAndrew, Craig, and Robert B. Edgerton. 1969. *Drunken Comportment: A Social Explanation*. Chicago: Aldine.

Makar, Ol'ha. 2014. "Volonteri maidanu Liza Shaposhnik ta Vitaliy Popov odruzhilisya v subotu" [Maidan volunteers Liza Shaposhnik and Vitaly Popov married on Saturday]. *Ukrainska Pravda*, May 24. http://life.pravda.com.ua/person/2014/05/24 /169563/.

Mars, Sarah G., Jason N. Fessel, Philippe Bourgois, Fernando Montero, George Karandinos, and Daniel Ciccarone. 2015. "Heroin-Related Overdose: The Unexplored Influences of Markets, Marketing and Source-Types in the United States." *Social Science and Medicine* 140 (September): 44–53.

Mason, Katherine. 2016. *Infectious Change: Reinventing Chinese Public Health after an Epidemic*. Stanford, CA: Stanford University Press.

Mattick, Richard P., Courtney Breen, Jo Kimber, and Marina Davoli. 2009. "Methadone Maintenance Therapy Versus No Opioid Replacement Therapy for Opioid Dependence." In *Cochrane Database of Systematic Reviews*. John Wiley. http://onlinelibrary .wiley.com/doi/10.1002/14651858.CD002209.pub2/abstract.

———. 2014. "Buprenorphine Maintenance versus Placebo or Methadone Maintenance for Opioid Dependence." *Cochrane Database of Systematic Reviews*, no. 2 (February): CD002207. https://doi.org/10.1002/14651858.CD002207.pub4.

Matza, Tomas. 2014. "The Will to What? Class, Time, and Re-Willing in Post-Soviet Russia." *Social Text* 120: 1–10.

McLaughlin, Daniel. 2015. "New Kiev Patrol Force the Beginning of Police Reform." *Irish Times*. May 22. http://www.irishtimes.com/news/world/europe/new-kiev-patrol -force-the-beginning-of-police-reform-1.2221493.

Metro.co.uk, Metro Reporter for. 2016. "Drug Dealer Whipped with Cable Ties and 'Beaten to Death.'" *Metro* (blog), February 16. http://metro.co.uk/2016/02/16/drug -dealer-whipped-with-cable-ties-and-beaten-to-death-5685325/.

Meyers, Todd. 2013. *The Clinic and Elsewhere: Addiction, Adolescents, and the Afterlife of Therapy*. Seattle: University of Washington Press.

Mimiaga, Matthew J., Steven A. Safren, Sergiy Dvoryak, Sari L. Reisner, Richard Needle, and George Woody. 2010. "'We Fear the Police, and the Police Fear Us': Structural and Individual Barriers and Facilitators to HIV Medication Adherence among Injection Drug Users in Kiev, Ukraine." *AIDS Care* 22 (11): 1305–13.

Ministry of Health of Ukraine. 2015. "Nakas MOZ Ukrayiny vid 03.27.2012 № 200 'Pro zatverdzhennya poryadku provedennya zamisnoyi pidtrymuval'noyi terapiyi khvorikh z opioyidnoyu zalezhnistyu'" [Order 200 of the MoH of Ukraine, enacted March 27, 2012, 'On regulations for the provision of substitution therapy for those with opioid dependence']. http://www.moz.gov.ua/ua/portal/dn_20120327_200.html.

Mitskaniuk, V. V. 2000. "Vnedreniye konseptsii snizheniya vreda v gorode Cherkasse" [The introduction of the concept of harm reduction in the city of Cherkassy]. *Zhurnal mikrobiologii, epidemiologii i immunobiologii*, no. 4 (August): 103–5.

Morozova, Olga, Sergey Dvoriak, Iryna Pykalo, and Frederick L. Altice. 2017. "Primary Healthcare-Based Integrated Care with Opioid Agonist Treatment: First Experience from Ukraine." *Drug and Alcohol Dependence* 173 (April): 132–38.

Moscow Times. 2014. "Poroshenko Challenged to Duel by East Ukrainian Rebel Leader." November 19. https://themoscowtimes.com/news/poroshenko-challenged-to-duel-by-east-ukrainian-rebel-leader-41525.

Mukharji, Aroop, and Vera Mironova. 2017. "Vera Mironova on ISIS Drinking, Embedding in Conflict Zones, and the Job Market for Insurgents." Podcast. Harvard Belfast Center: Office Hours. https://soundcloud.com/harvard/vera-mironova-on-isis-drinking-embedding-in-conflict-zones-and-the-job-market-for-insurgents.

Murney, Maureen Ann. 2009. "Mores of Addiction: Alcohol, Femininity, and Social Transformation in Western Ukraine." (PhD diss., University of Toronto, Canada).

Nabatov, Alexey A., Olga N. Kravchenko, Maria G. Lyulchuk, Alla M. Shcherbinskaya, and Vladimir V. Lukashov. 2002. "Simultaneous Introduction of HIV Type 1 Subtype A and B Viruses into Injecting Drug Users in Southern Ukraine at the Beginning of the Epidemic in the Former Soviet Union." *AIDS Research and Human Retroviruses* 18 (12): 891–95.

National Institute on Drug Abuse. 2016. "The Science of Drug Abuse and Addiction: The Basics." https://www.drugabuse.gov/publications/media-guide/science-drug-abuse-addiction-basics.

Nemtsova, Anna. 2014. "Ukraine Rebels Love Russia, Hate Gays, Threaten Executions." *Daily Beast*, October 25. https://www.thedailybeast.com/articles/2014/10/25/ukraine-rebels-love-russia-hate-gays-threaten-executions.

New York Times. 2014. "Ukraine Provides Evidence of Russian Military in Civil Unrest." April 20. https://www.nytimes.com/interactive/2014/04/20/world/europe/ukraine-provides-evidence-of-russian-military-in-civil-unrest.html.

Newman, Dina. 2015. "Ukraine Crisis: What Is Novorossiya Role?" *BBC News*, February 16. http://www.bbc.com/news/world-europe-31490416.

Nguyen, Vinh-Kim. 2010. *The Republic of Therapy: Triage and Sovereignty in West Africa's Time of AIDS*. Durham, NC: Duke University Press.

Nichter, Mark. 1989. "Pharmaceuticals, Health Commodification, and Social Relations: Ramifications for Primary Health Care." In *Anthropology and International Health*, 233–77. Culture, Illness, and Healing 15. Netherlands: Springer.

Ong, Aihwa. 2006. *Neoliberalism as Exception*. Durham, NC: Duke University Press.

Orcau, Àngels, Joan A. Caylà, and José A. Martínez. 2011. "Present Epidemiology of Tuberculosis: Prevention and Control Programs." *Enfermedades infecciosas y microbiologia clinica* 29 Suppl 1 (March): 2–7.

Ostrovsky, Simon. 2015. "Selfie Soldiers: Russia Checks in to Ukraine." VICE News, June 16. https://news.vice.com/video/selfie-soldiers-russia-checks-in-to-ukraine.

Owczarzak, Jill. 2009. "Defining HIV Risk and Determining Responsibility in Postsocialist Poland." *Medical Anthropology Quarterly* 23 (4): 417–35.

Owczarzak, Jill, Mikhail Karelin, and Sarah D. Phillips. 2015. "A View from the Frontlines in Slavyansk, Ukraine: HIV Prevention, Drug Treatment, and Help for People Who Use Drugs in a Conflict Zone." *International Journal of Drug Policy* 26 (1): 6–7.

Page, J. Bryan, and Merrill Singer. 2010. *Comprehending Drug Use: Ethnographic Research at the Social Margins*. New Brunswick, NJ: Rutgers University Press.

Parfitt, Tom. 2004. "Global Fund Suspends Payments to Ukraine." *The Lancet* 363 (9408): 540. https://doi.org/10.1016/S0140-6736(04)15580-3.

Parran, Theodore V., Joseph Z. Muller, Elina Chernyak, Chris Adelman, Christina M. Delos Reyes, Douglas Rowland, and Mykola Kolganov. 2017. "Access to and Payment for Office-Based Buprenorphine Treatment in Ohio." *Substance Abuse: Research and Treatment* 11 (June). https://doi.org/10.1177/1178221817699247.

Parsons, Michelle A. 2014. *Dying Unneeded: The Cultural Context of the Russian Mortality Crisis*. Nashville, TN: Vanderbilt University Press.

Parsons, Talcott. 1951. *The Social System*. Glencoe, IL: Free Press.

Patico, Jennifer. 2008. *Consumption and Social Change in a Post-Soviet Middle Class*. Stanford, CA: Stanford University Press.

Peacock, Elizabeth. 2012. "The Authentic Village and the Modern City: The Space-Time of Class Identities in Urban Western Ukraine." *Anthropology of East Europe Review* 30 (1): 213–36.

Pertsev, Andrey. 2017. "The Beginning of the End of Russia's Power Vertical." Carnegie Moscow Center. January 31. http://carnegie.ru/commentary/67848.

Petryna, Adriana. 2002. *Life Exposed: Biological Citizens after Chernobyl*. Princeton, NJ: Princeton University Press.

Petryna, Adriana, and Karolina Follis. 2015. "Risks of Citizenship and Fault Lines of Survival." *Annual Review of Anthropology* 44 (1): 401–17.

Pfeiffer, James, and Rachel Chapman. 2010. "Anthropological Perspectives on Structural Adjustment and Public Health." *Annual Review of Anthropology* 39 (1): 149–65.

Phillips, Sarah D. 2008. *Women's Social Activism in the New Ukraine: Development and the Politics of Differentiation*. Bloomington: Indiana University Press.

———. 2010. *Disability and Mobile Citizenship in Postsocialist Ukraine*. Bloomington: Indiana University Press.

Pinkham, Sophie. 2016. *Black Square: Adventures in Post-Soviet Ukraine*. New York: W. W. Norton.

Plokhy, Serhii. 2017. *The Gates of Europe: A History of Ukraine*. New York: Basic Books.

Polonets, V. V., and L. I. Andrushchak. 2000. "Sovmestnaya rabota NGO i UNAIDS po realizatsii proyekta po profilaktike VICH / SPIDa sredi lyudey, upotreblyayushchikh narkotiki putem in'yektsiy v regione s otnositel'no nizkim urovnem rasprostraneniya VICH-infektsii" [The joint work of NGOs and UNAIDS in realizing a project for the prevention of HIV/AIDS among people using narcotics by injection in a region with relatively low rates of HIV infection spread]. *Zhurnal mikrobiologii, epidemiologii i immunobiologii*, no. 4 (August): 92–93.

Prokhanov, Aleksandr. 2014. "Kto ty, 'Strelok'?" [Who are you, Strelkov?] *Zavtra*, November 20. https://web.archive.org/web/20151022094126/http://zavtra.ru/content/view/kto-tyi-strelok/.

Pulitzer Center. 2014. "Crimea: The Human Toll." Pulitzer Center. September 17. http://pulitzercenter.org/projects/europe-ukraine-crimea-russia-human-rights-LGBT.

Putin, Vladimir. 2005. "Annual Address to the Federal Assembly of the Russian Federation." Moscow, April 25. http://en.kremlin.ru/events/president/transcripts/22931.

Rachkevych, Mark. 2014. "Armed Pro-Russian Extremists Launch Coordinated Attacks in Donetsk Oblast, Seize Regional Police Headquarters, Set up Checkpoints (UPDATE)." *KyivPost*, April 12. https://www.kyivpost.com/article/content/war-against-ukraine/armed-pro-russian-extremists-seize-police-stations-in-donetsks-slavyansk-shaktarysk-fail-to-take-donetsk-prosecutors-office-343195.html.

Raikhel, Eugene. 2010. "Post-Soviet Placebos: Epistemology and Authority in Russian Treatments for Alcoholism." *Culture, Medicine and Psychiatry* 34 (1): 132–68.

———. 2013. "Placebos or Prostheses for the Will? Trajectories of Alcoholism Treatment in Russia." In *Addiction Trajectories*, 188–212. Durham, NC: Duke University Press.

———. 2016. *Governing Habits: Treating Alcoholism in the Post-Soviet Clinic*. Ithaca, NY: Cornell University Press.

Rasell, Michael. 2013. "Poverty and Social Welfare in Eastern Europe, Russia and Central Asia." In *Eastern Europe, Russia and Central Asia 2014*, edited by D. Heaney. Vol. 14e. The Europa Regional Surveys of the World. Europa Publications/Routledge (Psychology Press).

Rausing, Sigrid. 2014. *Everything Is Wonderful: Memories of a Collective Farm in Estonia*. New York: Grove Press.

Reid, Anna. 1997. *Borderland: A Journey through the History of Ukraine*. Boulder, CO: Westview.

Reuters. 2013. "Shaposhnik Works inside an Improvised Kitchen at Independence Square in Kiev." Thomas Reuters Foundation News. December 21. http://news.news.trust.org/item/20131221092548-4k2op.

Rhodes, Lorna A. 1996. "Studying Biomedicine as a Cultural System." In *Medical Anthropology: Contemporary Theory and Method*, 165–80. Westport, CT: Praeger.

Richardson, Tanya. 2008. *Kaleidoscopic Odessa: History and Place in Contemporary Ukraine*. Toronto: University of Toronto Press.

Rivkin-Fish, Michele R. 2005. *Women's Health in Post-Soviet Russia: The Politics of Intervention*. Bloomington: Indiana University Press.

Roache, Madeline. 2017. "Russia's Methadone Ban Is Fueling an HIV Epidemic in Crimea." November 11. http://themoscowtimes.com/articles/russias-methadone-ban-is-fueling-a-hiv-59488.

Robins, Steven. 2006. "From 'Rights' to "Ritual: AIDS Activism in South Africa." *American Anthropologist* 108 (2): 312–23.

Rose, Nikolas. 2007. *The Politics of Life Itself: Biomedicine, Power, and Subjectivity in the Twenty-First Century*. Princeton, NJ: Princeton University Press.

Rosenblum, Daniel, Fernando Montero Castrillo, Philippe Bourgois, Sarah Mars, George Karandinos, Jay Unick, and Daniel Ciccarone. 2014. "Urban Segregation and the US Heroin Market: A Quantitative Model of Anthropological Hypotheses from an Inner-City Drug Market." *International Journal of Drug Policy* 25 (3): 543–55.

"Rossiskaya Federatsiya Federal'nyy zakon o narkoticheskikh sredstvakh i psik-hotropnykh veshchestvakh" [Russian Federation federal law on narcotic drugs and psychotropic substacnes]. 1998. http://base.consultant.ru/cons/cgi/online.cgi?req =doc;base=LAW;n=154942.

Rubchak, Marian J. 1996. "Christian Virgin or Pagan Goddess: Feminism versus the Eternally Feminine." In *Women in Russia and Ukraine*, edited by Rosalind Marsh, 315–31. Cambridge: Cambridge University Press.

Sackett, D. L., W. M. Rosenberg, J. A. Gray, R. B. Haynes, and W. S. Richardson. 1996. "Evidence Based Medicine: What It Is and What It Isn't." *BMJ: British Medical Journal* (Clinical Research Ed.) 312 (7023): 71–72.

Scheper-Hughes, Nancy, and Margaret M. Lock. 1987. "The Mindful Body: A Prolegomenon to Future Work in Medical Anthropology." *Medical Anthropology Quarterly* 1 (1): 6–41.

Schoen, Doug. 2014. "Video Proof of Russian Military in Ukraine Emerges." *Forbes*, August 24. http://www.forbes.com/sites/dougschoen/2014/08/26/video-proof-of-russian -military-in-ukraine-emerges/.

Segalov, Michael. 2015. "The Number of Russian Troops Killed or Injured Fighting in Ukraine Seems to Have Been Accidentally Published." August 26. https://web.archive .org/web/20150826134411/http://www.independent.co.uk/news/world/europe/the -number-of-russian-troops-killed-or-injured-fighting-in-ukraine-seems-to-have-been -accidentally-published-10472603.html.

Shevchenko, Daryna. 2014. "EuroMaidan Protester Who Won Hearts Finds Her One True Love." *KyivPost*, June 5. https://www.kyivpost.com/article/guide/people /euromaidan-protester-who-won-hearts-finds-her-one-true-love-350811.html.

Shuster, Simon. 2013. "The World's Deadliest Drug: Inside a Krokodil Cookhouse." *Time*, December 5. http://time.com/3398086/the-worlds-deadliest-drug-inside-a -krokodil-cookhouse/.

Singer, Merrill, and Hans Baer. 1995. *Critical Medical Anthropology*. Amityville, NY: Baywood.

Singer, Merrill, and J. Bryan Page. 2014. *The Social Value of Drug Addicts: Uses of the Useless*. Walnut Creek, CA: Routledge.

Skryzhevska, Liza, Dávid Karácsonyi, and Kateryna Botsu. 2014. "Separatism in Donbas in the Context of Ukraine's Regional Diversity." *Perspectives on Europe* 44 (2): 50–62.

Snyder, Timothy. 2012. *Bloodlands: Europe Between Hitler and Stalin*. New York: Basic Books.

Solomon, Susan Gross. 1989. "David and Goliath in Soviet Public Health: The Rivalry of Social Hygienists and Psychiatrists for Authority over the Bytovoi Alcoholic." *Soviet Studies* 41 (2): 254–75.

Sonne, Paul, and Philip Shishkin. 2014. "Pro-Russian Commander in Eastern Ukraine Sheds Light on Origin of Militants." *Wall Street Journal*, April 26. https://www.wsj .com/articles/SB10001424052702304788404579526160643349256.

Sontag, Susan. 1988. *AIDS and Its Metaphors*. New York: Farrar, Straus and Giroux.

Spicer, Neil, Daryna Bogdan, Ruairi Brugha, Andrew Harmer, Gulgun Murzalieva, and Tetiana Semigina. 2011. "'It's Risky to Walk in the City with Syringes': Understanding Access to HIV/AIDS Services for Injecting Drug Users in the Former Soviet Union Countries of Ukraine and Kyrgyzstan." *Globalization and Health* 7: 22. https://doi.org /10.1186/1744-8603-7-22.

Spradley, James. 1970. *You Owe Yourself a Drunk: An Ethnography of Urban Nomads*. Boston: Little, Brown.

Star, Susan Leigh, and James R. Griesemer. 1989. "Institutional Ecology, 'Translations' and Boundary Objects: Amateurs and Professionals in Berkeley's Museum of Vertebrate Zoology, 1907–39." *Social Studies of Science* 19 (3): 387–420.

Starks, Tricia. 2008. *Body Soviet: Propaganda, Hygiene, and the Revolutionary State*. Madison: University of Wisconsin Press.

Steglenko, Dmitry. 2015. "V Krymu v resul'tate spetsoperatsii pogib sotrudnik FSKN" [Officers of the National Drug Control Service killed in special operations in Crimea]. *CrimeaMedia*, December 19. http://crimeamedia.ru/glavnoe/918-v-krymu-v-rezultate -specoperacii-pogib-sotrudnik-fskn.html.

Stillo, Jonathan. 2015. "'We Are the Losers of Socialism!'" *Anthropological Journal of European Cultures* 24 (1): 132–40.

Stuckler, David, Sanjay Basu, Martin McKee, and Lawrence King. 2008. "Mass Incarceration Can Explain Population Increases in TB and Multidrug-Resistant TB in European and Central Asian Countries." *Proceedings of the National Academy of Sciences of the United States of America* 105 (36): 13280–85. https://doi.org/10.1073/pnas .0801200105.

Szabo, Ross. 2011. "Has Peace Corps Become Posh Corps? Comparing Volunteers Then and Now." *Huffington Post* (blog), June 30. http://www.huffingtonpost.com/ross-szabo /peace-corps-posh-corps_b_887566.html.

Talavera, Oleksandr. 2015. "5 Reasons Why Ukraine's Crimea Is Happy With Russia." *VoxUkraine* (blog), January 5, 2015. https://voxukraine.org/en/happy_crimea_happy_russia/.

Taylor, Adam. 2014. "'Novorossiya,' the Latest Historical Concept to Worry about in Ukraine." *Washington Post*, April 18. https://www.washingtonpost.com/news /worldviews/wp/2014/04/18/understanding-novorossiya-the-latest-historical-concept -to-get-worried-about-in-ukraine/.

Tomkiw, Lydia. 2016. "Russia-Ukraine Conflict: Two Years after Crimea Annexation, Region Is a 'Black Hole' for Human Rights." *International Business Times*, March 19. http://www.ibtimes.com/russia-ukraine-conflict-two-years-after-crimea-annexation -region-black-hole-human-2338629.

TSN. 2014. "Na Donbasse terroristy mobiliziruyut narkomanov i alkogolikov: Seleznev" [They are recruiting addicts and alcoholics in Donbas: Seleznev]. TSN.Ua. June 17. https://ru.tsn.ua/politika/na-donbasse-terroristy-mobiliziruyut-narkomanov-i -alkogolikov-seleznev-371863.html.

Ukraine News One. 2014. "Donetsk Gay Club Attacked by Separatists (VIDEO)." *KyivPost*, June 10. https://web.archive.org/web/20140610164330if_/http://www.youtube .com/embed/vJ7bZ4XJjX4?rel=0.

"Ukraine Seeks Foreign Help on Police Reform." 2015. Bloomberg.Com. February 5. http://www.bloomberg.com/news/articles/2015-02-05/ukraine-seeks-foreign-help -on-police-reform.

UNAIDS. 2015. "Ukraine Harmonized AIDS Response Progress Report: Reporting Period: January 2012–December 2014." Geneva. http://www.unaids.org/sites/default /files/country/documents/UKR_narrative_report_2015.pdf.

———. 2016. "Ukrainian Government to Fully Finance Opioid Substitution Therapy." November 3. http://www.unaids.org/en/resources/presscentre/featurestories/2016 /november/20161103_ukraine.

———. 2018. "Ukraine | UNAIDS." http://www.unaids.org/en/regionscountries/count ries/ukraine.

U.S. President's Emergency Plan for AIDS Relief. 2013. "Ukraine: Operational Plan Report FY 2013." http://www.pepfar.gov/documents/organization/222186.pdf.

———. 2017. "Ukraine Country Operating Plan (COP) 2017: Strategic Direction Summary." https://www.pepfar.gov/documents/organization/272024.pdf.

———. 2018. "Ukraine Country Operating Plan (COP) 2018: Strategic Direction Summary." https://www.pepfar.gov/documents/organization/285850.pdf.

Valverde, Mariana. 1998. *Diseases of the Will: Alcohol and the Dilemmas of Freedom.* Cambridge: Cambridge University Press.

Verdery, Katherine. 1996. *What Was Socialism, and What Comes Next?* Princeton, NJ: Princeton University Press.

———. 1999. *The Political Lives of Dead Bodies: Reburial and Postsocialist Change.* New York: Columbia University Press.

Vickerman, P., N. K. Martin, and M. Hickman. 2013. "Could Low Dead-Space Syringes Really Reduce HIV Transmission to Low Levels?" *International Journal of Drug Policy* 24 (1): 8–14.

Voice of Russia. 2014. "Intoxicated Riot: Even Ukrainian Side Admits Use of Drugs in Kiev Maidan." May 16. http://voiceofrussia.com/2014_05_16/Intoxicated-riot-even -Ukrainian-side-admits-use-of-drugs-in-Kiev-Maidan-2223/.

Volkow, Nora. 2006. "Drug Addiction: Neurobiology of Disrupted Free Will." Presented at the Clinical Center Grand Rounds, Bethesda, MD, December. https://videocast.nih .gov/Summary.asp?File=13553&bhcp=1.

———. 2015. "Addiction: A Disease of Free Will." Presented at the Annual Meeting of the American Psychiatric Association, Toronto. https://www.drugabuse.gov/videos/dr -nora-volkow-addiction-disease-free-will.

Wakeman, Sarah E., Traci C. Green, and Josiah D. Rich. 2014. "From Documenting Death to Comprehensive Care: Applying Lessons from the HIV/AIDS Epidemic to Addiction." *American Journal of Medicine* 127 (6): 465–66.

Walker, Shaun. 2011. "Krokodil: The Drug That Eats Junkies." *The Independent*, June 22. http://www.independent.co.uk/news/world/europe/krokodil-the-drug-that-eats -junkies-2300787.html.

———. 2015. "Ukrainian Drug Addicts Dying Due to Treatment Ban, Says UN." *The Guardian*, January 20. https://www.theguardian.com/world/2015/jan/20/ukrainian -drug-addicts-dying-due-to-treatment-ban-says-un.

——. 2016. "Crimean Tatars Accuse Russia of Kidnappings and Political Arrests." *The Guardian*, December 12. https://www.theguardian.com/world/2016/dec/12/crimean-tatars-accuse-russia-of-kidnappings-and-political-arrests.

Wanner, Catherine. 2010. *Burden of Dreams: History and Identity in Post-Soviet Ukraine.* University Park: Penn State University Press.

Warner, Michael. 2002. "Publics and Counterpublics (Abbreviated Version)." *Quarterly Journal of Speech* 88 (4): 413–25.

Washington Post. 2014. "Transcript: Putin Says Russia Will Protect the Rights of Russians Abroad." March 18. https://www.washingtonpost.com/world/transcript-putin-says-russia-will-protect-the-rights-of-russians-abroad/2014/03/18/432a1e60-ae99-11e3-a49e-76adc9210f19_story.html.

Weaver, Courtney. 2014. "Ukraine's Rebel Republics." *Financial Times*, December 5. https://www.ft.com/content/9f27da90-7b3f-11e4-87d4-00144feabdc0.

Welsh, Christopher, and Adela Valadez-Meltzer. 2005. "Buprenorphine." *Psychiatry* 2 (12): 29–39.

Werf, Marieke J. van der, O. B. Yegorova, Nelly Chentsova, Y. Chechulin, E. Hasker, V. I. Petrenko, J. Veen, and L. V. Turchenko. 2006. "Tuberculosis-HIV Co-Infection in Kyiv City, Ukraine." *Emerging Infectious Diseases* 12 (5): 766–68.

World Health Organization (WHO). 1992. *International Statistical Classification of Diseases and Related Health Problems (10th Revision).* Geneva: Author. http://www.who.int/classifications/icd/en/.

——. 2004a. "WHO/UNODC/UNAIDS Position Paper: Substitution Maintenance Therapy in the Management of Opioid Dependence and HIV/AIDS Prevention." http://apps.who.int/iris/bitstream/10665/42848/1/9241591153_eng.pdf?ua=1.

——. 2004b. "Treating Tuberculosis in Ukraine." May 11. http://www.who.int/features/2004/tb_ukraine/en/.

——. 2005. "Ukraine: Summary Profile for HIV/AIDS Treatment Scale-Up." http://www.who.int/hiv/HIVCP_UKR.pdf.

——. 2010. "WHO Model List of Essential Medicines (March 2010)." Geneva: Author. http://www.who.int/medicines/publications/essentialmedicines/en/index.html.

——. 2012. "Evidence Based Medicine Related Resources." http://apps.who.int/rhl/education/Education_EBM/en/index.html.

——. 2015. "WHO | Dependence Syndrome." http://www.who.int/substance_abuse/terminology/definition1/en/.

World Health Organization (WHO) Regional Office for Europe. 2013. "HIV/AIDS Treatment and Care in Ukraine: Evaluation Report." http://www.euro.who.int/__data/assets/pdf_file/0004/194071/Evaluation-report-on-HIV-AIDS-treatment-and-care.pdf.

——. 2017. "Tuberculosis Country Brief, 2016: Ukraine." http://www.euro.who.int/__data/assets/pdf_file/0004/335542/UKR_TB_Brief_0223-AM-edits-D1-20-03-17.pdf?ua=1.

Yankovskyy, Shelly. 2016. "Political and Economic Transformations in Ukraine: The View from Psychiatry." *Transcultural Psychiatry* 53 (5): 612–29.

Yekelchyk, Serhy. 2014. "From the Anti-Maidan to The Donbas War: The Spatial and Ideological Evolution of the Counter Revolution in Ukraine (2013–2014)." *Perspectives on Europe* 44 (2): 63–69.

Yurchak, Alexei. 2008. *Everything Was Forever Until It Was No More*. Princeton, NJ: Princeton University Press.

Zalati, O., A. Iatsiuk, and T. Nepomniashchaia. 2000. "[The introduction of projects to prevent HIV infection among people using injection narcotics and women in the sex business in the city of Simferopol']." *Zhurnal mikrobiologii, epidemiologii i Immunobiologii*, no. 4 (August): 106–8.

Zhukova, Viktoriya. 2013. "Radicalizing Europe: Transnational and National Dimensions of Biopolitics, Health and HIV/AIDS. The Case of Ukraine." Budapest, Central European University.

Zigon, Jarrett. 2010. *"HIV Is God's Blessing": Rehabilitating Morality in Neoliberal Russia*. Berkeley: University of California Press.

Zinets, Natalia. 2014. "More than 40 Killed in Fire, Clashes in Ukraine's Odessa." *Reuters*, May 2. https://www.reuters.com/article/us-ukraine-crisis-odessa-fire/at-least-four-ukrainians-killed-in-odessa-violence-building-set-on-fire-idUSBREA410RP20140502.

Zinoviev, Alexander. 1985. *Homo Sovieticus*. Boston: Atlantic Monthly Press.

"'Zombie Apocalypse' in Russia: Krokodil Drug Turns People into 'Zombies.'" 2012. *International Business Times*, August 9. http://www.ibtimes.com/zombie-apocalypse-russia-krokodil-drug-turns-people-zombies-742607.

Zule, William A. 2012. "Low Dead-Space Syringes for Preventing HIV among People Who Inject Drugs: Promise and Barriers." *Current Opinion in HIV and AIDS* 7 (4): 369–75.

Index

Note: Page references in italics indicate illustrations; page references with an n indicate notes.

CPSIA information can be obtained
at www.ICGtesting.com
Printed in the USA
LVHW091803260619
622433LV00001B/138/P